WHY SHOULD YOU STOP SMOKING?

Cigarette smoking presents very real hazards to your health. In 1993, lung cancer surpassed breast cancer as the number one cancer killer among women. Numerous other diseases, such as heart disease, stroke, and emphysema are linked to cigarettes as well.

Your cigarette smoking puts your loved ones and friends in danger. Secondhand smoke has been proven to contribute to respiratory diseases in children, spouses, family members—anyone who lives with the smoker.

WHAT THIS BOOK OFFERS:

- help in figuring out when and where to quit: on a regular day? over a weekend? during a vacation?

- help in deciding which method will be the most successful for *you:* cold turkey? gradual cessation? with nicotine replacement?

- a discussion of the often-underestimated societal pressures on women to keep smoking

- clearly outlined strategies for alleviating withdrawal symptoms

- ways to overcome mental gremlins that rationalize having "just one cigarette"

- an invaluable chapter telling how to prevent relapse and giving three simple ways to overcome it

Quitting smoking is hard for anyone, but women face unique biological and societal challenges. If you are simply thinking about quitting, *or* if you are ready to quit and ready to work hard, *How Women Can Finally Stop Smoking* will help you, as a woman, find the best way to stop.

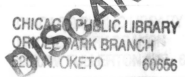

ABOUT THE AUTHORS

Robert C. Klesges, Ph.D., is a clinical psychologist. He is a Professor of Psychology at Memphis State University as well as a Professor of Preventive Medicine at the University of Tennessee, Memphis. He has published over one hundred scientific articles on health promotion in general and smoking cessation in particular. He has spoken at universities, medical centers, and national conferences throughout the country on smoking cessation techniques for women. Since 1983, his research on smoking has been funded by the National Institutes of Health. Dr. Klesges lives in Memphis with his wife, Lisa, and their son, Christopher, with another child on the way.

Margaret DeBon, M.S., is a doctoral candidate at Memphis State University. For the past five years she has held positions on grant-supported study teams investigating chronic obstructive pulmonary disease, Alzheimer's disease, and smoking cessation. In the past few years she has worked almost exclusively on women's issues and women and smoking cessation, publishing scientific articles in these areas.

ORDERING INFORMATION

HOW WOMEN
Finally
CAN STOP
∧
SMOKING

ROBERT C. KLESGES, Ph.D.
and Margaret DeBon, M.S.

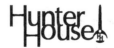

Hunter House Inc., Publishers
P.O. Box 2914
Alameda, CA 94501-0914

The authors are grateful for permission received to reprint from the following: *We
Are Still Married* by Garrison Keillor, NY: Dutton Inc., © 1989, used by permission
of the publisher; the graph on page 22 from *Cancer Facts and Figures*, American
Cancer Society, 1990.

Library of Congress Cataloging-in-Publication Data

Klesges, Robert C.
How women can finally stop smoking / Robert C. Klesges and Margaret DeBon.
1st ed.   p. cm.
Includes bibliographical references and index.
ISBN 0-89793-147-5: $8.95
1. Women—Tobacco use. 2. Cigarette habit—Treatment. 3. Self-help techniques.
I. DeBon, Margaret. II. Title.
RC567.K56 1993
613.85'082—dc20   93–41456

Copyeditor: Rosemary Wallner   Proofreader: Susan Burckhard
Cover design: Beth Hansen   Book design: *Qalagraphia*
Project Editor: Lisa E. Lee   Production Manager: Paul J. Frindt
Marketing: Corrine M. Sahli   Promotion: Robin Donovan
Customer Support: Laura O'Brien, Sharon Olson, Sergio Gaspari, James Rachogan
Fulfillment: A & A Quality Shipping Services
Publisher: Kiran S. Rana

Typeset by 847 Communications, Alameda CA
Printed and bound by Griffin Printing, Sacramento CA
Manufactured in the United States of America

9 8 7 6 5 4 3 2 1   First edition

CONTENTS

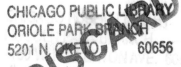

FOREWORD

Smoking is responsible for over 400,000 deaths in the United States in 1990. This addiction already causes one-third of all cancer deaths and over half of heart attack deaths in women, but it has an even more profound effect on them. The 40 different carcinogens identified in cigarette smoke wreak havoc on the immune systems of both men and women, and there are effects on women's reproductive tracts that are well documented yet poorly publicized. Smoking increases a woman's risk of infertility, ectopic pregnancy, and miscarriage. Once a woman become pregnant, her smoking causes higher rates of premature delivery and sudden fetal death. The baby of a smoker has a lower birth weight, and a higher chance of dying during the time around birth. It has also been shown that women who smoke have higher rates of abnormal pap smears and cervical cancer. This is because the toxins from smoking are absorbed into the bloodstream and carried to distant organs. Research reveals that women who smoke develop urinary incontinence more often. Smoking women also have been shown to lose calcium from their bones at a much faster rate than nonsmokers, causing higher rates of osteoporotic fractures, and slower healing. Interestingly, smoking seems to decrease a woman's blood levels of estrogen, both before menopause and after menopause, even when she takes hormone replacement therapy. Some research suggests that smoking can increase a woman's risk of breast cancer during menopause.

These facts are not well-known, and that is a feminist issue. Why a feminist issue? We must recognize that there are indeed inherent differences between men and women. These differences can be exploited and misused, as in the cigarette advertising campaigns to recruit women to smoke, which started in the early 1960s, creating images of smoking women as having more freedom, popularity, and success. Later cigarette brands were created very specifically for women which were longer, more slender, and more "feminine." Some brands even linked their cigarettes to the women's movement with slogans such as, "You've come a long way, baby," and portrayals of defiant women with cigarettes rising above the societal proscription against women smoking, showing dazzling strength and character.

These effective campaigns have taken their toll on women. The lung cancer rate for women in 1960 was only six per 100,000, and steadily rose to 28 per 100,000 by 1987, and continues to increase. In 1979, lung cancer became the greatest killer of women, above even breast cancer, and persists today in taking the lives of over 50,000 women annually. We women have been exploited and used. While there exist strong efforts to limit smoking in public places, and to make smoking socially unacceptable, no one of these efforts succeeds in undoing the effects of the media in recruiting women to smoke.

Quitting smoking carries immediate as well as long-lasting benefits. Lung function improves and risks of heart attack and stroke decline soon after your last cigarette is smoked. These risks largely dissipate after two to three years of not smoking. Yet quitting smoking has been described as much more difficult than even quitting heroin, and has finally received the attention of the National Institute of Drug Abuse, which had previously focused only on illegal drug use and addiction. Recognizing the national death toll from cigarettes, this agency is focusing on their powerful addictive potential, calling tobacco a fatally addictive drug, whose producers are the only industry in the United States whose products are causally associated with the deaths of its users when the products are used as directed. As many as 60–90% of smokers want to cut down or quit, but can't because of the addictive properties of cigarettes.

Smoking *is* a feminist issue. The exploitation of women by the media must stop, but it will only stop if it is proven ineffective. We can make it ineffective by not smoking and by not allowing our friends and colleagues to smoke. The "tough love" therapy of the groups who deal with narcotics addiction can teach us to actively support our associates in giving up the habit and choosing health. The psychological messages underpinning all addictions are that the individual lacks the strength, the self-concept, or the moral drive to have good health. Feminism is only about the health and well-being of women. The message of feminism is that, in fact, we are very strong, deserve to have strong self-concepts, and have the moral strength to live a very healthy life. This serves not only the women we know but also those who learn from us, our families, our world, and tomorrow's world.

This wonderful and effective book derives not simply from the facts we know about smoking, but in a major and important way from the facts we know about *women*. This book is tailored to women's unique skills and strengths, geared to overcome their most common pitfalls in successfully conquering a serious addiction, and creating a long-lasting focus on health. The authors have incorporated scientific information about concerns most women have which hinder the quitting process, such as weight gain and social support. They draw from a very lengthy and broad experience in running their own clinic specifically for women, which boasts a very high success rate for both quitting and staying off of tobacco. They recognize the *process* of smoking cessation and take their clients and you, the reader, beyond that last puff into a healthier life.

As a cancer specialist, I must say it breaks my heart repeatedly to see my patients die of avoidable and preventable cancers. It is never appropriate at a time of diagnosis to explain to a cancer patient that her cancer was entirely avoidable, but most women will volunteer that they know their smoking caused their current state. In my practice, I never stop asking patients to quit smoking. Some of them leave me and see other doctors who won't bother them so. But I see my role as promoting only good health, and am grateful to have such a good tool for helping women create this important change in their life. Thank you Dr. Klesges and Ms. DeBon! Thank you from all women!

Katherine A. O'Hanlan, M.D.
Associate Director, Gynecologic Cancer Section
Stanford University School of Medicine

ACKNOWLEDGMENTS

The authors would like to thank both of our families for their patience and support during the late nights we worked on this book. We would also like to thank William Applegate, M.D., M.P.H., for his helpful comments on Chapter 4 and Andrew Meyers, Ph.D. for his years of guidance with our program at Memphis State. Finally we would like to thank the National Heart, Lung, and Blood Institute of the National Institutes of Health for supporting our research efforts over the years.

AN IMPORTANT
NOTE TO THE READER

The material in this book is intended to provide an overview on the issues surrounding women and cigarettes and a guide for women stopping smoking. Every effort has been made to provide accurate and dependable information and the contents of this book have been compiled in consultation with other professionals. However, you should be aware that professionals in the field may have differing opinions, and change is always taking place. The publisher, authors, and editors cannot be held responsible for any error, omission, professional disagreement, or outdated material. If you have any questions or concerns about the information in this book, please consult a licensed health practitioner.

Because of new research, changes in government regulation, and the continuing flow of information related to nicotine replacement therapy, you are advised to consult your physician and the package insert for nicotine replacement for the latest information. The authors and publisher disclaim any liability for loss, injury, or damage incurred as a direct or indirect consequence of the use and application by you of these materials, individually or in consultation with a professional or group.

The persons and events described in the interviews in this book are real, but their names have been changed to protect their privacy.

INTRODUCTION

If you are a woman who wants to learn more about smoking, this is the book for you. It doesn't matter whether you are ready to quit smoking or not. You don't even need to be thinking seriously about quitting. Let us explain why.

There are different stages of change women go through when they quit smoking. You, as a woman smoker, most likely are at one of three stages.

First, there are women who are not yet ready to quit. If you are this type of smoker, quitting smoking may be the furthest thing from your mind. You know smoking is bad for you, but you aren't ready to think about quitting smoking.

If you are like most women who smoke, you are in the second stage: you are thinking about quitting, but aren't sure when you will do it. You probably say things like, "I know I should quit, but. . . ." (fill in the rest yourself: my job is too stressful, I don't want to gain weight, I'm concerned about withdrawal symptoms, etc.) You want to quit, but you aren't ready to make the serious effort to quit and stay quit.

Finally, there are those of you who are ready to quit. You have gone through the above stages and are ready to make a serious quit attempt. (You really shouldn't try to quit unless you are ready to make a serious attempt.)

No matter what stage you are at, there are two major reasons you should read this book. First, as we discuss in the Introduction, this is the first smoking book designed for the unique needs of the woman smoker. We know that women start smoking, continue to smoke, and quit smoking for different reasons than men. There are unique things women can do that will help you quit and things you need to pay particular attention to. Second, we wrote this book to help you, the woman smoker. Since you have to go from one stage to another to successfully quit, we designed this book to help you no matter which stage you are currently in.

When you do quit smoking, it will probably by be one of the more difficult things you will ever do. It will also be one of the most important things you will ever do for you and the people around you. Start down that road today.

SUCCESS FOR WOMEN

*"Why does my wife need special attention
to help her quit smoking?"*
—the husband of a smoker enrolled
in our stop-smoking program

This question is one we hear often and raises a valid point. Women would need a unique program only if they smoked (and quit) for different reasons than men.

Our research team at the Prevention Center at Memphis State University has been studying women and smoking for eight years. We have treated thousands of women smokers. We have talked to those who have successfully quit smoking as well as those who have failed. We have researched several aspects of women and smoking, publishing over 50 scientific articles on this topic. Members of our research team have contributed to three Surgeon General's reports on the health consequences of smoking. We have constantly changed, modified, and improved our stop-smoking program based on our research as well as the research of others.

What have we learned from all this research and clinical experience? For one thing, we know that there are differences between why women smoke and why men smoke. Additionally, women quit smoking for different reasons than men. Most importantly, we now know there are specific and different things that will help women quit smoking . . . and stay quit.

This book was written to help women quit smoking whenever they are ready. It is based on the stop-smoking programs that we conduct in Memphis, Tennessee. Smoking cessation researchers have taught us much about generic, effective strategies for quitting smoking (for example, monitoring intake before quitting and setting a quit day). In this book, we have combined their best, most effective strategies and added specific strategies for women.

We have divided this book into two parts. The first part discusses the facts we feel every woman needs to know before she quits smoking. We discuss influential people and groups (largely cigarette companies) that have a vested interest in your smoking habit.

The second part is a step-by-step guide to quitting (and staying off cigarettes). First, we discuss nicotine replacement (the patch and nicotine gum) and help you determine if that approach is right for you. Then we help you prepare yourself for quitting, which includes cutting down on the number of cigarettes you currently smoke. We discuss the quit day and what to do (and not to do). We talk about overcoming mental gremlins and preventing unwanted post-cessation weight gain. Most importantly, we talk about staying quit. A quote often ascribed to Mark Twain sums up how some people feel about quitting: "Quitting smoking isn't hard; I've done it several thousand times." The key is not just to quit, but to stay quit.

HOW TO USE THIS BOOK

If you are not yet ready to quit but would like more information about smoking, read Part I. Since Part II is devoted to the nuts and bolts of quitting, you will not need to read this section until you are ready to make a cessation attempt. Reading Part I provides you with information that will motivate you to think more about trying to quit.

If you are thinking about quitting but are not sure about when, read Chapters 1 through 5. Once you are ready to set a quit date, read through the rest of the book.

If you are ready to quit, we recommend that you read the entire book. The information presented in Part I will encourage you as you quit. Pay close attention to the information in Chapter 4 on nicotine replacement.

Occasionally at our stop-smoking program, women will tell us that they don't need to be convinced about quitting. They will say they have decided to use nicotine replacement and are ready to quit smoking. They will tell us they only need help with how to quit.

If you are at this point, you might want to begin your reading with Part II. Part I will help work through *why* you should quit. Part II will tell you about nicotine replacement along with *how* to quit. Read and reread the sections that pertain to where you are right now.

The numbers in parentheses in the text refer to endnotes, found on page 165. Because of the controversial nature of some of this material, we have noted major sources of references for anyone interested in further research.

Nobody can force you to do something that you don't want or aren't ready to do. In our stop-smoking program when less-than-motivated subjects fail to quit in our program, the most common complaint is that we didn't "make" them quit smoking. We can't *make* you stop smoking—we can't *make* you do anything. However, if you are ready to quit and work hard, this book will help.

PART I

WHAT YOU NEED TO KNOW
BEFORE YOU QUIT SMOKING

1

HOW MEN AND WOMEN DIFFER IN THEIR SMOKING

You may think you are alone, one of the last cigarette smokers around. You have tried to quit and may know many people who have done so successfully. Your family and/or your spouse or partner are pressuring you to stop smoking. You feel guilty and want to quit but don't think you can.

Do any of these people sound like you or anyone you know?

> *Elaine:* "I've tried to quit several times. My husband quit several years ago. I don't know what's wrong with me. I'm just a weak person."

> *Heather,* age 16: "I started smoking last year. It makes me feel cool. And it really helps me watch my weight."

> *Suzanne:* "Everybody else has quit. All my friends have quit. You can't smoke anywhere anymore. I must be the only cigarette smoker left in town."

> *Jan:* "If I quit smoking, maybe I'll live longer. It'll sure *seem* longer."

Despite trying to quit several times, *Elaine* is still smoking. Since she tried to quit and failed, she concluded that she is weak. If this has happened to you, you need to know that—according to the American Cancer Society—women may be less likely to quit smoking than men.(1) National research (including our own) has shown that women begin to smoke for different reasons than men, they quit for different reasons than men, and they relapse for different reasons as well.

As *Heather*, an adolescent smoker, points out, smoking makes you feel cool. She strongly believes that smoking helps control her body weight—she's right, it does—but not as much as people think. Heather is just one of millions of adolescent girls who are taking up the habit. The U.S. Department of Health and Human Services has found that adolescent girls are generally more likely to start smoking than adolescent boys. This trend has held true for several years. Meanwhile, rates for men have been steadily declining over the past years and boys, in general, do not seem eager to take up the habit. Girls, however, are beginning to smoke in greater numbers than before. In fact, rates have been *increasing* in recent years.(2)

Suzanne, who is older, feels alone. She perceives herself as the "only cigarette smoker left in town." Indeed, newspaper articles, television shows, and even cartoons lead us to believe that no one is smoking any longer. It seems like smokers *can't* smoke anywhere anymore. Garrison Keillor pokes fun at the image of the lone smoker in his short story, "End of the Trail:"

> The last cigarette smokers in America were located in a box canyon south of Donner Pass in the High Sierra by two federal tobacco agents in a helicopter who spotted the little smoke puffs just before noon.... The five smokers were handcuffed and transported to a federal detention camp in Oregon, where they were held in pup tents for months.

There is real truth in Suzanne's belief. Rates of smoking are generally down. Large numbers of men have quit; in the past 20 years, the rates of smoking among men are down over 50 percent.(3) However, rates of smoking among women have not declined over the past 20 years. The American Cancer Society estimates that by the turn of the century there will be more women smoking than men.

Jan knows that smoking is bad for her health, yet that isn't enough to make her want to quit. Because women are smoking more than ever, women's health is suffering. The American Heart Association says that rates of heart attacks, strokes, and other cardiovascular diseases have decreased less in women than in men. Emphysema, which is largely due to smoking, and other lung problems have also stayed relatively unchanged over recent years. However, if you are like most women, your biggest health fear is not heart or lung disease—it's cancer. And while cancer of any kind is scary, you are probably most fearful of breast cancer. Did you know that the number one cause of cancer death in this country among women is no longer breast cancer? In a 1992 report, the American Cancer Society said that lung cancer is now the number one killer. Ten thousand more women die of lung cancer every year than of breast cancer. If you are diagnosed with breast cancer, your chance of being alive five years later is about 77 percent. If you get lung cancer, the chance of being alive for five years is only about 20 percent. And smoking is to blame.

WHY AREN'T WOMEN QUITTING SMOKING?

Why aren't women like you quitting smoking? Are women not informed about the health consequences of smoking? No, women know as much if not more about the health consequences of smoking as men. The vast majority of smokers, including women, indicate they want to stop smoking.(4) Are women really, as Elaine thinks, "weak individuals?" Of course not! From our research, and studies conducted by other smoking researchers in the United States, we now know that women are not quitting for seven important reasons.

Smoking makes you feel good

Nicotine is a highly addictive substance. In the 1988 *Surgeon General's Report on Smoking and Health*, Surgeon General C. Everett Koop declared cigarette smoking as addicting as heroin and cocaine. That is not to say that you are a "smoke addict" like a crack or heroin addict. Although smoking is highly addictive, the reasons why it is so pleasurable are different than for alcohol, heroin, or cocaine. Smoking is rewarding because it only takes about ten seconds from the beginning of a puff for nicotine to reach the brain.(5) The quicker one receives pleasure, the more rewarding the experience. That is why oral amphetamines, which typically take over 30 minutes to take effect, are much less addictive than crack cocaine, which reaches the brain almost immediately.

Not only does nicotine act quickly, it makes us feel better. Many smokers report that smoking helps them concentrate and lifts their mood. Several studies, including one done in 1988 by the U.S. Department of Health and Human Services, show improvement in attention, reaction time, and problem-solving abilities after smoking. Smokers commonly report pleasure and reduced anger, tension, depression, and stress after smoking.

Smokers report that cigarettes not only stimulate but also relax them. While this sounds like a contradiction, there is evidence to support this claim. Nicotine is known as a biphasic drug—it stimulates at lower levels and depresses at higher levels.(6) Early in the morning, when nicotine levels are at their lowest, you probably inhale deeper and slower to get more nicotine into your system. The low levels of nicotine tend to stimulate you, helping you to get going. As the day progresses into evening, your nicotine levels may increase to the point where further smoking may relax you. In other words, nicotine stimulates you when you want to be stimulated and relaxes you when you want to be relaxed.

Because of the many pleasurable aspects of nicotine, our program for women works on reducing nicotine intake so you can avoid many of the negative withdrawal symptoms associated with smoking. In Chapter 4 we discuss the relative advantages and disadvantages of the patch and nicotine gum.

Some stop-smoking programs downplay the reasons why people smoke. Some may even tell you that there is nothing about smoking that is rewarding and that everything about quitting is wonderful. We don't believe in this strategy. First, smoking *is* rewarding—if it weren't, you wouldn't be doing it. We believe that if you know what the barriers to quitting are and what attracts you to smoking, you will be better equipped to confront your habit and overcome it. We think that one of the biggest mistakes we in the health profession can make is to not inform people about their health status (for example, not telling a person how serious a medical illness is). If you are fully informed, at least you know what you are up against.

Smoking is something you do automatically . . . and a lot

Have you ever been engrossed in a book or movie and looked down at the ashtray after a couple of hours to see several cigarette butts—cigarettes you don't remember smoking? Smoking is automatic; we do it without thinking. We tend to put our cigarettes in the same spot, smoke in the same places (for example, in a favorite chair), and even use the same ashtrays, cigarette lighters, and matchbooks. In general, the more automatic the habit, the harder it is to break.(7) If you have ever tried to change a habit, whether it be nail biting, saying an overused phrase, or smoking, you know how tough it can be.

Not only is smoking automatic, it is something we do a lot. If you smoke one pack of cigarettes per day and inhale 15 times per cigarette, that is 109,500 inhalations per year. There are few things that you do that often. You don't eat, sleep, drink, have sex, or even have that many conversations in a year. This makes smoking a difficult habit to give up.

Because smoking is so automatic, our program systematically works on raising your *awareness* of smoking. We also teach you ways to give up something you do that has become a part of your daily life.

Smoking has become your best friend

Another reason for continued smoking is that it gives us pleasure and comfort in a wide variety of circumstances and settings. We have learned to associate smoking with drinking and alcohol or coffee, talking with friends, driving, finishing a meal, talking on the phone, and relaxing after sex. You may think that if you quit smoking, you will no longer enjoy alcohol, coffee, talking, driving, eating, and sex.

You shouldn't worry, however. You will continue to enjoy these activities after you quit smoking. Although you have learned to associate these activities with smoking, there is nothing inherent in smoking that makes these activities more pleasant. Think back to the first time you smoked: it was probably an unpleasant experience and, in all likelihood, you got sick. Because you *learned* to associate fun and pleasure with smoking, you can *unlearn* this association and these activities will be just as pleasant as before.

If you are like most woman smokers, smoking, in a way, has become sort of a friend, even a part of your personality. Like a friend, smoking is always there for you. It perks you up when you're blue; it's part of your daily life. Our program addresses these important issues, particularly in the first couple of days of not smoking. However, for now, just realize that smoking really isn't your best friend. Your best friend wouldn't try to kill you.

Quitting is short-term pain, long-term gain

One of the real problems when you quit smoking is that the pain associated with quitting is as immediate as the pleasures of smoking. Within 24 hours of quitting, you are likely to experience withdrawal symptoms.(8) Most withdrawal symptoms diminish significantly within two weeks—they are at their peak after one week—and you return to normal within a month. (9) Unfortunately, if you are unsuccessful in your attempts and resume smoking soon afterwards, you will alleviate your withdrawal symptoms and have to start the cycle all over again.

The pay-off for dealing with withdrawal is substantial— quitting increases the likelihood that you will live up to eight years longer. However, since many smokers who are trying to quit have not yet contracted a smoking-related disease, the concept of living longer is not always a powerful motivator, especially to someone who is going through tough withdrawal symptoms. As Elaine said after her relapse: "It was two o'clock in the morning, I couldn't sleep, and all I could think of was a cigarette. I didn't care if I didn't live until morning, I wanted a cigarette that bad."

Quitting smoking is difficult. If it were easy, you probably wouldn't be smoking. Indeed, most smokers say they would quit smoking if an easy method of quitting were offered to them. The worst thing we can tell you is that quitting smoking will be easy. While for a few people it *is* easy, the vast majority of smokers find it difficult to quit. If a smoking program offers you a guaranteed way to quit smoking without effort or withdrawal symptoms, the people running the program are probably either ignorant or are deceiving you (or put more bluntly, are fools or liars).

To illustrate our point, we know of a stop-smoking program that uses the slogan "Quitting Is Easy." What messages are they giving you when they tell you quitting smoking is easy? They tell you to expect success and that quitting is effortless. But when you try to quit, you find it difficult and become confused. You relapse. Most people *do* relapse the first time they quit smoking. In fact, most smokers try to quit an average of four times before they actually succeed.(10) You tried to quit, found it difficult, and started smoking again. But the program said it was easy! If you are like most women, you will probably blame yourself for this failure. Like Elaine, you may feel guilty, helpless, and weak. These feelings, in turn, may reduce the chances that you will quit again in the future. In fact, the blame should be placed on the program that told you to expect that quitting would be effortless.

Our program focuses on short-term goals and ways of motivating you to resist the urge for a cigarette. Research has taught us much about how and why women relapse. We emphasize simple strategies for avoiding relapse. We provide strategies that will help you even during the worst periods, and if you follow our three simple rules of relapse (see Chapter 8) you should be able to overcome most relapse situations.

Not everyone wants you to quit

As we discuss in Chapter 3, not everyone wants you to quit smoking. The cigarette industry and, to a lesser degree, other smokers encourage women to smoke. Although broadcast smoking advertisements have been banned in the United States for many years, pro-smoking messages brought to you by cigarette companies suggest that smoking will make you sexier, more popular, slimmer, more independent, and more able to enjoy yourself. They bombard us with these messages from billboards, newspapers, magazines, and at sporting events. Cigarette companies know that women are the ones smoking and are targeting their advertising toward you as a result. While men have one or maybe two "male" cigarettes (Marlboro, Camel), women have many (Virginia Slims, Capri, Eve, and others). Cigarette advertisements in women's magazines far exceed the ads for other products.

In our program we spend considerable time discussing the images that cigarette companies project of smokers, how these companies manipulate us, and how they encourage young people to start smoking. Despite their arguments to the contrary, there is evidence that cigarette companies are trying to get young women to start smoking and are encouraging adult women to continue to smoke.(11) If Chapter 3 gets you mad at the cigarette companies, good. Perhaps we can collectively put these companies out of business.

Smoking controls body weight

Probably the biggest single difference between men and women smokers is that women are much more concerned about post-cessation weight gain than men. Several early smoking programs tried, with good intentions, to downplay the weight gain associated with smoking cessation. A commonly cited statistic is that one-third of smokers gain weight, one-third stay the same weight, and one-third lose weight.(12) This statistic means that two-thirds of smokers have nothing to worry about when they quit.

Wouldn't it be wonderful if this were true? But based on your own experience, you probably already know that this statistic is wrong. Actually, 75–80 percent of smokers *do* gain weight (approximately five pounds) when they quit smoking, while the remainder stay the same weight. Unfortunately, while women are most concerned about post-cessation weight gain, they are also more likely than men to gain weight.

Smoking programs have not addressed the special needs of women smokers

Are you aware that many of the stop-smoking programs popular today are based on research that was conducted, in some cases, decades ago? No real new methods, other than the patch and nicotine gum, have been developed in the past several years.(13) Consequently, many of the most effective programs were tested—and confirmed—with male participants. This is not too surprising since 20 years ago most of the smokers were men, and men were much more likely to die of smoking-related disease.

Smoking cessation programs (indeed, many health promotion programs) in the early days relied on two basic assumptions. The first was that if sizable numbers of smokers quit, we would observe large reductions in lung cancer, emphysema, and heart disease. This assumption was correct. Along with this reduction of smoking, we have observed a large reduction in smoking-related disease (particularly heart disease) among men.

The second assumption was that if programs could be used successfully with white men, they would also be successful with women, minorities, and those with low incomes. Unfortunately, this assumption was incorrect, particularly with women. Today, there is evidence that women may be less likely to attempt cessation, and they are more likely to relapse after they quit.(14) If you, like Elaine, feel alone and frustrated because you can't quit, be assured that millions of women have probably experienced what you are going through.

But you and Elaine *can* quit. With your commitment and our strategies, you can address the issues that keep you smoking and keep you from quitting.

EIGHT THINGS YOU
SHOULD DO TO STOP SMOKING

We have found eight keys to women's success, and they form the basis of our program. We will introduce them here, and explain how they work in the following chapters.

Watch your cycle when deciding when to quit

In recent years, several research studies have shown that smoking and the menstrual cycle interact. A number of symptoms associated with the menstrual cycle are identical to those of smoking withdrawal. These include irritability, anxiety, hunger, and decreased concentration. It is possible that women smokers mistake normal menstrual symptoms with those of smoking withdrawal. Another possibility is that menstrual symptoms may combine with withdrawal symptoms and become intolerable.

Both smoking withdrawal symptoms and menstrual symptoms increase in the premenstrual or latter part of the cycle and during your period. Recently collected data from our lab suggests that it is harder for a woman to quit smoking in the premenstrual phase of her cycle or during her period than right after her period. Therefore, plan to quit at the end of your period (the beginning of your cycle); you will experience fewer and less intense withdrawal symptoms.

Reduce your caffeine consumption

If you are like most smokers, you drink caffeinated beverages such as coffee, tea, or soft drinks. Researchers have found that women who smoke are more likely to drink caffeinated beverages than women who don't smoke.(15) There is much confusion about what to do with your caffeine intake; many women wonder if they should increase or decrease it. Some programs advocate eliminating caffeine altogether because drinking the beverage will remind you of smoking. Some stop-smoking counselors recommend that you increase your caffeine intake. They reason that caffeine will act as a substitute stimulant for cigarettes, which also have stimulant qualities.

Research suggests, however, that you should reduce your caffeine intake by about half. As it turns out, cigarette smoking reduces caffeine's effects. As a smoker, you need almost twice as much caffeine as a nonsmoker to get the same effect.(16) When you quit smoking, your body normalizes its response to caffeine. If you don't reduce your intake, you might experience symptoms of a caffeine overdose, such as nervousness, irritability, and tension. These symptoms, like menstrual symptoms, can either mimic or add to smoking withdrawal symptoms.

Team up with a friend

Studies have shown that the social support provided by the buddy system is related to successful smoking cessation in women.(17) Interestingly, social support has little or no effect on cessation in men. However, there are pitfalls with the buddy system, which is only as good as its weakest link. We will talk about the right and wrong types of social support and how to choose the right buddy for you in Chapter 5.

Recognize the differences between men who smoke and women who smoke

Women may have a harder time quitting smoking than men. Although there are a number of behavioral reasons for this, there appears to be a biological reason as well. Women seem to metabolize nicotine slower than men.(18) This may mean that, cigarette for cigarette, women may have higher nicotine levels than men. This could make women more nicotine dependent and make the process of quitting much more difficult because of more intense withdrawal symptoms. While research in this area is preliminary, it provides one possible explanation why women find it difficult to quit smoking.

Cut down first

For men, the question of whether to cut down or quit cold turkey may not matter. For women, however, cutting down first is important. Because women metabolize nicotine slower, they may experience more intense withdrawal symptoms, and are more likely to report symptoms of increased eating and weight gain than men.(19) Chapter 5 includes a section on cutting down before you quit.

Recognize your mental gremlins

It is common for women to internalize and blame themselves when they fail to quit. If you are like most women, you have tried at least once to quit smoking and have relapsed. It is likely that you experienced some negative emotion along with this relapse. Some women feel guilty; others become depressed or angry at themselves. Many conclude that they are weak or inadequate, and their feelings of self-worth and self-esteem typically take a beating.

This process is known as experiencing negative emotions or negative affects. Statements pop into our heads that drive these negative emotions. We like to describe these automatic thoughts as mental gremlins, those self-defeating ideas that may prompt a relapse. Examples of mental gremlins are:

"What will one cigarette hurt?"

"Everything kills you these days. Why should I quit smoking? It's just one of a million things that will hurt you."

"I'm going to die from something anyway. Besides, I could get hit by a car tomorrow. At least this way, I know what's going to get me."

The first gremlin tells you to go ahead and have a cigarette—because you will stop at just one. (While it is possible to stop at just one, it is unlikely.) The second and third gremlins allow you to rationalize your habit by minimizing the health consequences of smoking or adopting a fatalistic view. You can imagine the result of listening to these gremlins.

Mental gremlins are predictive of relapse; women have both more intense and a greater number of gremlins than men do. We will discuss mental gremlins in more detail in Chapter 7.

Learn the facts about quitting smoking and weight gain

Few people want to gain weight. However, most people do gain weight when they quit smoking and, unfortunately, women are more likely to gain weight than men.(20) Fortunately, our own research efforts, as well as those of others, have identified many of the reasons why women gain weight when they quit smoking. Additionally, we have researched both behavioral strategies and pharmacologic aids, such as nicotine gum, for reducing post-cessation weight gain. We focus on these strategies in Chapter 9.

Confront relapses

Many women believe that smoking is an either/or proposition. Either you are a smoker or you are not. To paraphrase an effective quote from Alcoholics Anonymous, many smokers believe that "one cigarette is too much; a million cigarettes are never enough." That is, one slip, one cigarette, and you are back to smoking.

There is no question that a single slip is predictive of relapse. However, women tend to do better in a smoking cessation program that is more oriented toward problem-solving and will help them mobilize their psychological forces and overcome relapses through long-term effort.(21) In contrast, men may be more successful using a "total abstinence" approach or one more in line with the "one cigarette is too much" philosophy. As such, our program is geared toward problem solving, which is most likely to be successful for women smokers.

With these keys to stopping smoking in mind, let's look at the effects of smoking—what it does to you and those around you. We bet that once you know the very real personal and social hazards, you will find more reasons and inspirations to stop.

2

WOMEN—YOUR LIFE
COULD BE GOING UP IN SMOKE!

Did you know that smoking is the number one cause of preventable death and disability in the United States? According to a 1992 study by the American Lung Association, as many as 500,000 people in the United States die of smoking each year. Every 20 months more people die of diseases caused by cigarette smoking than by combat in World War I, World War II, the Korean War, the Vietnam War, and the Gulf War *combined*. More people in the United States die from the diseases caused by cigarettes than from alcoholism, car accidents, homicides, suicides, and AIDS *combined*.

Imagine the tragedy of a plane crash that kills 58 people and permanently disables many others. Now imagine an airplane crashing every hour of every day—that's how many people in the United States die of diseases caused by cigarettes each year.

Up to one-third of all smokers will die prematurely of smoking-related ailments.(1) The next time you are with two other smokers, look to your left and then to your right—one of you will die from a disease caused by smoking. Those aren't very good odds, are they?

Most people think of lung cancer and emphysema when they think of smoking-related diseases. Indeed, about 90 percent of the incidences of lung cancer and most cases of emphysema are smoking-related. Smoking also increases the risk of heart disease and stroke. In 1993, the American Heart Association reported that at least 100,000 women smokers die each year from heart disease or stroke caused by their smoking.

Many women believe that only men develop heart disease and experience strokes. While it is true that younger men die of heart attacks and strokes more often than younger women, the rate of heart disease increases for women once they reach menopause. In fact, at that point, the risk of heart disease is actually higher in women than in men of the same age, according to the American Heart Association.

The good news is that you can undo most, if not all, of the harmful effects of smoking—even if you have smoked for years.

MORE BAD NEWS
ABOUT CONTINUING TO SMOKE

It may surprise you to learn that smoking rates among women may soon exceed the smoking rates of men.

Figure 1 shows the rates of smoking for men and women in the United States over the past 20 years. As you can see, the rate of smoking in men has decreased significantly. Among women, the rate has decreased only slightly. Given that the population is increasing, there are *more* women smokers in the United States today than there were ten years ago. It is estimated that by about the year 2000 there will be more women in this country than men.

In 1988, the U.S. Department of Health and Human Services reported that most surveys of teen smokers show that more girls than boys are beginning to smoke. The evidence even suggests that the *percentage* of girls who take up smoking is on the increase.

This high rate of smoking takes a tremendous toll on women's health. Figure 2 shows women's deaths due to lung

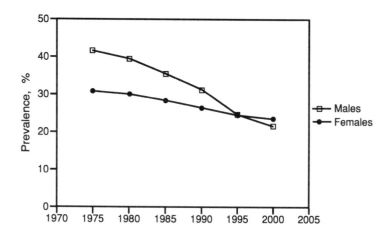

Figure 1   Smoking rates for men and women
over the past 20 years

Source: J.P. Pierce, M.C. Fiore, et al. (1989). Trends in cigarette smoking
in the United States: Projections to the Year 2000. JAMA, 261, 61–65.

and breast cancer over the past 40 years. In 1950, deaths due
to breast cancer in the United States were much greater than
deaths due to lung cancer. While deaths attributed to breast
cancer have risen only slightly over the past 40 years, the
number of deaths from lung cancer began to skyrocket around
1970. By 1987, lung cancer had outstripped breast cancer as a
leading cause of death for women. Since then, this trend has
continued. Each year, there are now 10,000 women who die
from lung cancer than breast cancer. The chances of surviving
breast cancer are *much* greater.

Smoking can be detrimental to health even when it isn't
deadly. Here are other health consequences of smoking:

- If you have problems sleeping, you can put part of the
  blame on smoking. At the 1993 meeting of the Associated Professional Sleep Societies, two professors reported on smokers and sleep. They concluded that

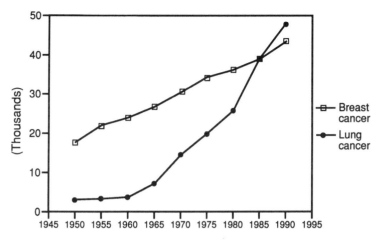

Figure 2   Women's death rates due to lung cancer and
breast cancer, 1950–1988

Source: American Cancer Society, 1990, Cancer Facts and Figures

smokers were twice as likely to have nightmares and nine times more likely to snore. They were more restless overnight and more likely to wake up tired. So smoking even hurts you when you sleep.

- People who smoke around young children expose them to environmental tobacco smoke (secondhand smoke), which is the worst kind of carcinogen and can cause cancer.(2) Secondhand smoke is the leading cause of respiratory problems and lowered pulmonary function (strength of the lungs) in infants and children.(3) Cigarette smoke also puts children at risk for middle ear infections, which is the leading cause for surgical hospitalization in young children.(4) Children who are exposed to their parents' smoke are two to four times more likely to die of Sudden Infant Death Syndrome than children who have nonsmoking parents.(5)

- The number of parents who smoke is a strong predictor of whether or not children smoke.(6)

- If you want to preserve your eyesight, quit smoking. A 1992 study has shown that smoking is associated with an increased incidence of cataracts.(7)

- Smoking causes skin wrinkles and premature aging.(8)

Also, smoking has some specific effects on women:

- Smoking increases the risk of many disorders that can prevent pregnancy. A smoker is more likely to become infertile and has a higher risk for ectopic pregnancies, a potentially life-threatening condition which occurs when the fertilized ovum implants itself in the cervix, fallopian tubes, ovary, or abdominal or pelvic cavity instead of the uterus.(9) The body almost always aborts ectopic pregnancies.

- Women who smoke while taking oral contraceptives greatly increase their risk of high blood pressure or other serious cardiovascular problems, including the probability of death from heart disease.(10) As the 1990 *Physician's Desk Reference* indicates, "Women who use oral contraceptives should be strongly advised not to smoke."

- Women who smoke have twice the incidence of pelvic inflammatory disease—any infection of the cervix, uterus, ovaries, or fallopian tubes—than women who don't smoke.(11)

- Even rates of osteoporosis—a reduction in bone density—are higher among smokers.(12) Osteoporosis is a common health hazard among postmenopausal women. Although there is currently no effective treatment for osteoporosis, studies show that it can be prevented by giving up smoking and by adding calcium to your diet.

- The average age of menopause is much younger among women who smoke.(13) Women smokers experience menopause anywhere from one to three years earlier than women who do not smoke.

- Smoking during pregnancy is strongly related to infant death prenatally and at birth.(14) Low birth weight is one of the best predictors of whether or not your baby has a serious, life-threatening medical complication. The more you smoke, the more likely your child will have a low birth weight.(15) Women who stop smoking prior to pregnancy or within the first three to four months reduce this risk so that is equivalent to that of a nonsmoker.(16)

As the cigarette ads claim, smoking does something special for women. However, that something "special" is all bad.

THE GOOD NEWS ABOUT QUITTING SMOKING

By now, you may be a bit depressed about all the dangers of cigarette smoking. If you are like many smokers, you may also be a bit scared and angry. When we teach our stop-smoking classes in Memphis, smokers commonly react by saying:

"I had no idea that smoking did all those things to me."

"I thought smoking was only hurting me; I didn't know it was hurting my kids."

However, there is some good news:

- You can literally "turn back the clock" if you quit smoking. If you quit smoking and do not get a smoking-related illness for about five years, you will live virtually as long as someone who never smoked!(17)

- Within 24 hours of quitting smoking, you decrease the probability of sudden death.

- You will gain years of life regardless of how many years you have smoked, how many cigarettes per day you smoked, or how old you are.(18) No matter what your age, it's never too late to quit smoking.

- Quitting smoking pays. Not only do you improve your health, you help your pocketbook. When you add up the price of cigarettes, insurance premiums, and burns in your clothes, smoking costs you at least $600 per year.(19) Imagine what you could do with that money.

- When you quit smoking your sense of smell and taste improve, breathing becomes easier, and you look and smell clean.

- By quitting smoking you will feel better about yourself. You will act as a healthy role model for your friends, relatives, and children.

You have everything to gain and nothing to lose by quitting smoking!

THE MENTAL GREMLINS
THAT KEEP YOU SMOKING

Given all the health problems, why do people continue to smoke? One reason is that certain "inner messages" encourage us to continue to smoke. We use the term "mental gremlins" for these automatic thoughts that have a strong impact on our emotions. These gremlins can promote continued smoking by giving us positive notions about smoking while minimizing its harmful effects.

Do any of these positive gremlins sound familiar?

"I enjoy that first cigarette in the morning with coffee."

"There's nothing in the world quite as nice at the end of the day as a glass of wine and a cigarette."

"I smoke because I like the taste."

Mental gremlins can also encourage relapse when we are trying to quit. These negative gremlins often voice themselves when we are either craving a cigarette or have just had a slip.

"I don't have the willpower to quit."

"I tried to quit last week. I started snapping at everyone. I had to start smoking again or I probably would have lost my job (or my husband/partner)."

"When I quit last time, I gained ten pounds in two months and ate everything in sight. There's no way I am going to quit and let *that* happen again."

"The last time I quit smoking, my family told me I was turning into a bitch . . . so they told me to go back to smoking."

Most women smokers we have treated have responded to messages like these. These gremlins are so related to women's smoking and, we believe, smoking relapse that Chapter 7 is entirely devoted to them.

Gremlins are often active, but they tend to be most active when women are at risk for relapse and when women are deciding whether or not they are going to try to quit smoking. Over the past several years, we have heard a large number of "you don't really want to stop smoking, do you?" gremlins, which try to convince you that the dangers of smoking aren't nearly as great as they really are. These gremlins tend to make light of the hard, cold, undeniable fact that smoking is likely to kill you. Typically, a mental gremlin starts out with "Yes, that may be true *but* . . . . " During our training in clinical psychology, we learned that if we want to find out what someone *really* feels, we ignore what they say before the "but."

Our research group has treated thousands of women smokers over the years. From this work, we have compiled a list of mental gremlins that encourage people to keep smoking—and included ways to counteract them. You might recognize some of them as things you or your smoking friends have said. Many of us actually believe some of these mental gremlins. But they are gremlins—and everyone knows that gremlins are products of the imagination.

"Yeah. We're all going to die of something, it might as well be from smoking!"

It's true. We are all going to die someday. And we will die of something. The issue is *when* and *how*. This gremlin seems to make sense (most gremlins do, at least on the surface). But think about it. Believing this gremlin is like believing that there's no point stopping at red lights because we are all going to die someday anyway.

You can live up to seven or eight years longer if you quit smoking. Take a moment to think back seven years. What were you doing then? Where did you live? Where were you working? Think of all the happy times you have had over the past seven years—all the things that you will remember for the rest of your life. Now imagine all those years gone. That's what smoking does to you.

"It seems like everything kills you these days. Why should I quit smoking—it's just one of millions of things that can kill you."

This gremlin is one that we, as health researchers, have helped to create. It seems that every week there is a new study telling us something is harmful. We are bombarded with stories of things we should and should not do. Additionally, there have been contradictory reports. First it was reported that regular coffee was bad for us, then it was reported that it wasn't. Most recently, another study concluded that decaffeinated coffee is bad for us. For years, we have heard that cholesterol is bad for us. Then in 1988, a report called for a redefinition of levels of high cholesterol.(20) Even handheld cellular phones have come under attack—they allegedly cause brain cancer!

No wonder people are confused. The only way to sort out the confusion is to look for consistency in the research literature. This may surprise you, but some published research is seriously flawed or the findings are the result of a fluke. That is, auto mechanics can botch a job, a brand new stereo out of the box can fail to work, and researchers also err every now and then. Also, once in a long while, you can flip a coin ten times and come up with heads every time. Sometimes when you study something, you come up with strange (and incorrect) findings due to pure chance.

There are two rules to follow when you read about some new health hazard. First, never rely on a single study to change your mind about something you should or should not do unless the evidence is extremely compelling. For example, there are hundreds of studies that have found that cholesterol is bad for you. You shouldn't change your mind because of one study that comes to a different conclusion. Second, never rely on a single case study, particularly if there is a lawsuit pending. All the media attention about handheld cellular phones resulted from one individual who died of brain cancer. This was a tragic case and maybe there was something to it. However, it is best to reserve judgment until more research is conducted.

What would it take to convince you that something is bad for you—a hundred studies? A thousand? A thousand studies showing that something harms you certainly would convince most people. How about over 60,000 studies? That's how many published reports researchers have written on the health consequences of smoking.

While many things endanger our health, most medical researchers agree about the "big three." That is, of all the things you should do to protect your health, there are two or three you should focus on first. And at the top of everyone's list is: Stop smoking. It accounts for more disease and disability than anything else.(21) The other two are controlling hypertension and controlling significantly elevated cholesterol. This is not to say that other things such as exercise won't lengthen your life, but start with these three. Or, as one person told us, "I know I'm a walking risk factor. I smoke, I drink, I eat too much, you name it, I probably have it. But I'm only going to change a couple of things. What should I do?" Number one is stopping smoking.

So, this gremlin—that *everything* is a health hazard—only appears correct on the surface. It is based on understandable confusion. You can do a lot of good for yourself if you, first, stop smoking and then make sure your blood pressure and cholesterol are in the normal range.

"I've been smoking for years. It's too late for me. I've done too much damage to my body."

This gremlin is flat out *wrong*. There is now evidence that no matter how old you are, you add years to your life if you quit smoking—even if you are in your seventies or eighties.(22)

"You know, the tobacco companies keep saying that there is not conclusive proof that smoking causes disease."

Technically, they are partially correct. The only way we could know for sure whether or not smoking causes disease is to randomly assign half of the adolescents in the United States to either smoke or not smoke. Those who were assigned to smoke had to smoke and those assigned to not smoke could not smoke. Obviously, this can't be done.

What's the next best thing? Well, we know from animal studies (where random assignment is possible) that smoking exposure causes the same health problems that are observed in humans. Also, thousands of human studies show that smoking is related to disease.

If you believe seat belts and air bags reduce death and injuries in car accidents, penicillin can kill infections, and fluoride reduces cavities, you are basing your belief on *less* evidence than there is for the link between smoking and disease. So, don't let the tobacco companies fool you—this stuff kills.

"I know all the facts, but doesn't everything in life involve risk?"

We agree, but don't be misled by this argument. It is true that if you stayed in bed all day, you would be statistically safer than if you took a shower. There is a statistical probability that you will fall and bump your head while showering. Driving to work, eating, and a score of other everyday functions expose you to risk. However, most of us choose to accept some risk as part of everyday life. We weigh the advantages of a certain activity (for example, driving so that we can work) against the small risk we take by engaging in these activities. The risks we are willing to accept vary from person to person. Most of us are not willing to experience the thrill of parachuting or bungee jumping because of the risk involved. Other people disagree and feel that the experience is worth the risk.

But there are risks and there are risks. Of all the things that can hurt you, kill you, and shorten your life, smoking leads the list. While scientists disagree and debate about the relative risk of certain things such as the health risks of coffee, virtually everyone—except those who work for tobacco companies—agreed with former Surgeon General C. Everett Koop when he said "Cigarette smoking is the single most important . . . factor contributing to premature mortality in the United States today."

"My uncle lived to be 100 and he smoked two packs of cigarettes per day. And then there are people like Andy Kaufman, a non-smoker, who died of lung cancer at age thirty-five."

Every smoker we have met either knows or has heard of some person who smoked large numbers of cigarettes and lived to a ripe old age. Many smokers will also report knowing of a non-smoker who died at a young age of lung cancer or heart disease. Not every smoker dies from a disease related to their smoking; and some nonsmokers die of lung cancer. We simply don't know all the causes of lung cancer. Andy Kaufman, a well-known comedian, may have gotten cancer because of exposure to secondhand smoke or some other toxin, or something could have just gone wrong with his body.

Health promotion is about probabilities, not certainties. That is, by smoking, you greatly increase the probability of developing heart disease or lung cancer. By quitting smoking, you greatly decrease the probability of developing heart disease or lung cancer.

Suppose you found out that it was dangerous to walk into a particular building because it could collapse (like a smoker's lungs). If you walked into the building, you would have a 90 percent probability of dying. If you stayed in the street, you would have only a 10 percent probability of dying. Now, there's a probability that if you go in the building you will be safe and if you stay in the street you will die, but what choice are you going to make? This is how you need to think about the decision you make with smoking.

A slightly different gremlin uses a combination of anger and denial. We suspect we will see more of this kind of gremlin as additional antismoking regulations are enacted and the tobacco companies fuel the fire of smokers' discontent. (If you don't believe that tobacco companies are encouraging a backlash of pro-smoking, read any issue of *Phillip Morris Magazine*.)

The anger and denial gremlin is nicely illustrated by a Letter to the Editor that appeared in the June 25, 1993, edition of *USA Today*:

> Have we smokers become the "Negroes" of the past who had to sit in the back of buses and were denied service by restaurants? I am 69 years old and have been smoking since I was 21. My 71-year-old sister has smoked since she was 16. My mother smoked for about 40 years and lived to be 82.

There are two issues here. The first is the argument of an oppressed minority—"I choose to smoke; back off!" Much self-destructive behavior can occur if you are led to believe that you are an oppressed minority and that your rights are being taken away. As we discuss in Chapter 3, the cigarette companies are trying to get you to buy into this belief. Don't let emotion overtake rationality or think with misdirected anger. In this case, it could kill you.

The issue the letter brings up is that many smokers live rich, long lives. However, as Dr. Victor Strecher of the University of North Carolina pointed out at a 1993 conference of the National Cancer Institute in Bethesda, Maryland, there is another way to look at the statistics on smoking and health. If the difference in average life span between smokers and non-smokers is seven years and if about one out of four people die prematurely of their smoking, then three out of four people who smoke will probably live as long as nonsmokers.(23) However, it also follows that one out of four smokers will die 28 years prematurely of the disease caused by their cigarettes. In other words, it is like Russian Roulette. Are you willing to engage in something where there is a one in four chance that you will die almost three decades before you should?

Let's say that you are about to go on a cross-country car trip. You ask a mechanic to check out your car. The mechanic tells you that there is a one in four chance that you won't make it to your destination. In fact, the problem with your car is so great that there is a one in four chance that you will die before you get there. Would you leave on your trip anyway?

We have never met anyone who would. This is a different way of looking at the statistics; it helps explain why some smokers live long lives but it also points out how *much* some smokers have to lose.

"I may smoke, but I watch my weight, am physically active, and I watch what I eat."

Sorry, but you don't reduce or undo the dangers of smoking by having an otherwise healthy lifestyle. As we mentioned above, stopping smoking should be the first healthy lifestyle change you make.

"I won't be smoking forever. I plan to quit sometime soon."

We haven't met many women smokers who plan to be smokers for the rest of their lives. We have never had a woman smoker tell us that she is going to smoke until she gets lung cancer and dies. If you are like most women, you plan to quit—if not today, someday.

Unfortunately, for many smokers, that "someday" doesn't come quickly enough or at all. Many smokers tell us, "I don't want to quit now. I'll quit within the next five years." When we talk to them five years later, they tell us, "I don't want to quit now. I'll quit within the next five years."

The problem is that you never know when that smoking-related disease will come along and tell you "time's up." A colleague of ours told us the following true story about his mother.

Mrs. Smith had been smoking for years. All her children had pleaded with her to quit smoking, particularly Richard, who was a cardiologist. She always said, "Son, you don't have me convinced. I'll quit someday, but not right now."

At age 65, Mrs. Smith had a heart attack that was related to her smoking. When told to quit, she said "I'll quit someday, but not right now."

At age 68, Mrs. Smith was diagnosed with cancer in one lung. The lung had to be removed. She was told to quit. She said, "I'll quit someday, but not right now."

At age 71, she had a mild stroke. Her son again pleaded with her to quit smoking. She said, "Son, you don't have me convinced. I'll quit someday, but not right now."

At age 72, she was diagnosed with cancer in the other lung and she was told she would die. As her son entered her hospital room, he found her staring at her cigarettes. She looked at her son and said "Son, I think you've finally got me convinced."

This story illustrates why there is no better time to quit than right now. While you may not be ready to quit for a while, don't put it off another five years.

"I figure you're going to go when you're supposed to go."

This is not a common gremlin, but we hear it from people who are fatalistic—those who believe that God or some spiritual/cosmic entity has already determined their lives (and/or their deaths). One cannot come up with hard proof, one way or the other, regarding this gremlin. Perhaps we are in control of our destiny; maybe we aren't. However, even if someone truly believed in this gremlin and if they lived in a house with lots of dynamite, we doubt they would be lighting matches.

"Cancer doesn't run in my family. Why should I worry about smoking?"

The vast majority of smoking-related deaths are not from cancer, but from heart disease.

A member of one of our stop-smoking groups told a counselor that she wasn't going to quit smoking. When he asked her why, she replied, "Because I won't get lung cancer. Lung cancer doesn't run in my family. " When he asked her if heart disease ran in her family, she said, "Oh, yes, my dad died of a heart attack at 44 and my mom died of a stroke at 56." "You and I need to have a little talk," the counselor said. When he told her about the relationship between heart disease and smoking, you could see her jaw drop. To this day, she does not smoke.

"Yeah, smokers in general die from smoking. But I can beat the odds."

Perhaps you can, but if we were betting, we would bet against you. Whenever we hear this gremlin, we are reminded of the movie *The Big Red One*. It's based on the true story of a group of World War II soldiers who never got hurt even though they saw a tremendous amount of combat. Yet, other squad members and their replacements were killed or maimed. One afternoon, one of the new replacements approached a member of the group and said something like, you know what they call this squad, don't you? The ghost squad. You guys never get hurt, but the replacements all get killed. You think I'll get killed?" The soldier looked at him and had a chilling response: "Why not? You someone special?"

The point is that no smoker knows with any degree of certainty whether or not she will die because of smoking. Why take the chance?

"I tried to quit once. I was miserable. I feel better when I smoke!"

In many ways, we can sympathize with this gremlin. The smoker who said this probably was miserable when she quit (we were when we quit). At least right now, she probably does feel better when she smokes—or she will for a while. Quitting smoking is best described as short-term pain, long-term gain.

Suppose you go to the doctor and she tells you there is something wrong with your heart. Then she says, "You have to go into the hospital for treatment. You'll be in some real pain for about two weeks. Then you have to do some exercises. You'll have to do them for about two to four weeks after getting out of the hospital, then it will get much better. The pain *will* flare up every now and then, sometimes for a year after treatment. However, I can guarantee that if you respond like most women, you will live years longer."

Would you take the doctor's advice and go for treatment? We have yet to meet a woman who wouldn't. Quitting smoking is just like this example except that your treatment is reading and following the instructions in this book. You will feel bad for a couple of weeks and then it will get much, much better. You will need to do your exercises which involve following the simple strategies for quitting and avoiding relapse outlined in Part II. With time, you will have to use your exercises less and less. However, every now and then the pain, which is really an urge to smoke, will flare up, and you will have to practice your exercises (or strategies). You need this treatment badly. For many of you, it's a matter of life and death.

3

NOT EVERYONE
WANTS YOU TO QUIT

We have discussed all the important reasons to stop smoking. We have also discussed how difficult it is to quit smoking and introduced the techniques you will learn to make the process easier. In this chapter, we will tell you about the forces at work that are trying to *keep* you smoking. Although some of your smoking friends may not discourage you from smoking, a group of business people is actively *encouraging* you to smoke. This group spends billions of dollars each year trying to manipulate you to continue to smoke—and to get others to begin smoking. These companies are trying to convince you that cigarette smoking is associated with high-style living, healthy activities (!), and professional success.(1) We conclude the chapter by describing the message you convey to people by continuing to smoke.

The information in this chapter will cut through your excuses, denials, and ignorance of the dangers of smoking. You are not going to like what you hear. This information will anger you. It will also empower you in your attempt to quit.

CIGARETTE COMPANIES ARE
GETTING AWAY WITH MURDER

Many years ago, several toy companies started selling cheap, highly desirable toys. These toys were loved by boys and girls alike. As long as they had them, they were happy.

After these toys had been on the market for several years, many children started dying. Scientists suspected that these toys were to blame. The toy companies stated emphatically that their toys had been "proven safe" when, in fact, their own studies showed that the toys were dangerous. Instead of informing the public that their studies pointed to a problem, they actively suppressed this information.

Even when children continued to die—about one every minute of every day—the toy companies said that there was no proof that their toys hurt children. They suggested that children who bought these toys were probably just "naturally clumsy."

Is this pure fantasy, something from the pages of a bad novel? No. Replace the "toy stores" with "cigarette companies" and the "toys" with "cigarettes" and you have a true story. Newspaper accounts of a 1992 court case report that a cigarette company had evidence—collected by its own scientists—that smoking causes cancer and other health problems. In the United States today, smoking kills approximately one person every minute of every day. And yet the formal policy of cigarette companies is that there is no conclusive evidence that smoking causes health problems. The companies conclude that the death and illness associated with smoking are probably due to the fact that those who choose to smoke are naturally less healthy.

Some people might say, "What do you expect? Tobacco companies are out to make a buck just like everyone else. They are no different from any other company. They will do anything to make a profit."

If this has been your opinion up till now, we suspect you will change it by the end of this chapter. We don't think that all (or even most) companies are nearly as unscrupulous as most cigarette companies. For example, during the Tylenol poisoning scare in the early 1980s, the Johnson & Johnson corporation acted honestly and swiftly. It informed the public of the tampering and potential danger. It did more than the government said it had to do. It recalled all Tylenol products and tested them for additional tainted pills (at a cost of millions). The company subsequently developed and pioneered the use of tamper-resistant containers. All of this was done in response to less than a dozen deaths; which is equivalent to about 10–15 minutes worth of cigarette-related deaths.

Another conclusion you may make by the end of this chapter is that anyone who works for the tobacco companies is a sleazeball.

While the product and the active manipulating of information may show no regard for people's lives, we are convinced that there are many fine people who work for tobacco companies or grow tobacco crops. Some may have no choice; it is either that or no job. Others rationalize their work. As the former head of the National Cancer Institute said, either cigarette company employees have to personally admit to killing millions of people or they have to conclude that the scientific evidence is flawed.

Cigarette manufacturers spend up to an estimated $2.5 billion per year in advertising and promotion.(2) While the companies can no longer buy broadcast time, they still manage to get much television exposure by advertising at sporting and other events. Cigarettes are the most advertised product in outdoor media, the second most advertised product in magazines, and the third most advertised product in newspapers.(3) All six major cigarette manufacturers were among the 100 companies with the highest advertising budgets in 1985.

Perhaps the cigarette companies feel they need to advertise because in the United States fewer people are smoking. After all, the cigarette companies currently lose about 2 million smokers per year either through smoking cessation or smoking-related deaths.(4)

For many years, the tobacco industry has claimed that the

purpose of its advertising is to promote brand loyalty and prevent brand switching in current smokers rather than recruit new smokers.(5) Yet, if this were the case, the cigarette companies would be spending an estimated $345 per smoker per year to convince only the 10 percent of smokers who switch in a year.(6) Because most cigarettes sold in the United States are marketed by six companies—and 70 percent by two companies, Philip Morris and R. J. Reynolds—most brand switching would be intracompany, negating any profits from this enormous advertising and promotional expenditure.(7)

In these advertisements, there is evidence that cigarette companies target young children, women, minorities (particularly African Americans and Hispanics), and blue-collar workers.(8) Although the cigarette companies deny that they target individuals at risk for smoking.(9) From a strict marketing standpoint, this claim makes no sense. One of the basic rules of advertising is to target your coverage to the people most likely to buy the product. Men typically buy power tools; when was the last time you saw an advertisement for power tools in *Redbook*? We doubt you will see many feminine hygiene products advertised in *Popular Mechanics*. Despite the insistence that tobacco companies don't target their advertising, let's look at the evidence that cigarette companies target children and women.

Cigarette companies want your children to smoke

Cigarette advertisements are common in publications with large teenage readerships. Cigarette advertising expenditures in *Glamour*, where a quarter of the readers are girls under eighteen, were $6.3 million in 1985. In *Sports Illustrated*, where one-third of the readers are boys under eighteen, they were $29.9 million in 1987.(10) Children have a high rate of recognition of cigarette advertisements. In high school students, a strong positive relationship exists between smoking and advertisement recognition.(11) The more students smoke, the higher their advertisement recognition.

The most blatant example of promoting cigarettes to children, particularly young children, is R. J. Reynolds Nabisco's use of Old Joe (Cool) the Camel. In fact, one study had a particularly chilling title: "Brand Logo Recognition by Children Aged 3–6 years: Mickey Mouse and Old Joe the Camel."(12) Researchers found that one of the most recognized logos was Old Joe. Just over 50 percent of the children recognized and correctly identified Old Joe. In contrast, only 25.3 percent recognized Cheerios, 21 percent NBC, and only 16.2 percent recognized IBM. Sadly, only 10 percent knew what the Surgeon General's warning was. By age 6, as many children recognized Old Joe as recognized the logo for the Disney Channel.

RJR Nabisco argued that these results were misinterpreted —Old Joe was directed at adults and the recognition in children was just an unintended byproduct of this advertising. Another recent study evaluated the degree of children's recognition of Old Joe compared with adults. The study assessed a sample of over 1,500 adults and children regarding their knowledge and recognition of the Old Joe logo. The results were clear—children were much more knowledgeable about Old Joe than the adults. Children were more likely to report prior exposure to Old Joe (98 vs. 72 percent), were better able to identify the type of product being advertised (97 vs. 67 percent), and were more likely to name the cigarette, Camel, by name (94 vs. 58 percent). This targeting has had a direct impact on what children smoke. Camel's share of the illegal children's cigarette market has increased from 0.5 percent to almost 33 percent. This translates into over $475 million in sales per year.(13)

Finally, the Tobacco Institute, an organization completely supported by 12 companies that manufacture cigarettes and other tobacco products, published an antismoking pamphlet entitled "Tobacco: Helping Youth Say No." According to the institute, a panel of "education experts and individuals involved on a day-to-day basis with young people" wrote the copy. Note here they don't say that these are smoking experts.

Any parent would qualify as an individual who is involved "on a day-to-day basis with young people." Curiously, this panel of "experts" also did not include a single Ph.D. or M.D., despite the fact that probably dozens of reputable smoking researchers (including us) would have donated their time to help write an antismoking manual meant for free distribution.

While the goal of an antismoking pamphlet is, on the surface, admirable, there is concern that the message may actually increase adolescent smoking.(14) For example, the pamphlet never mentions that there are health issues involved; rather, the copy states that young people are aware of the claims that smoking presents risk to one's health. The pamphlet emphasizes that smoking is an adult behavior and that it is illegal to smoke as an adolescent. One of the quickest ways to promote an activity in a slightly rebellious adolescent is to declare that the activity is for adults only and that to engage in the activity is against the law.

These efforts to get young people to smoke seem to be working. In the late seventies, with the introduction of Virginia Slims and its "you've come a long way, baby" campaign, there was a marked upswing in the number of young girls taking up smoking, as Dr. Gary Giovino of the Centers For Disease Control has noted. Recently, researchers have observed an increase in the number of boys beginning to smoke. This has coincided with the introduction of Joe Camel.

If there was ever any doubt about the cigarette companies' intent, Robert, one of the authors, became personally convinced while driving with his five-year-old son. The two passed a tobacco shop with a sign of Joe Camel in the window. His young son exclaimed, "Look, Dad. A new toy store!"

Cigarette companies want women to smoke

Since 1968, cigarette companies have released several cigarette brands marketed specifically for women. Of these, Virginia Slims, More, Eve, Satin, and Ritz have become extremely good sellers. The companies have also marketed extensions of other brands that target women, including Newport Slim Lights and Salem Slim Lights. As R.M. Davis, in *The New England Journal of Medicine*, pointed out back in 1987: "The cigarette paper and package are often designed to appeal to women. Eve has a flower design on its filter tip; Satin has a satin-like paper tip; and Ritz, billed as the first 'designer cigarette,' bears the logo of the fashion designer Yves St. Laurent on its package and filter tip."

That same year, *Advertising Age* reported on a Philip Morris campaign being test-marketed in Switzerland. The company was promoting the cigarette Star as a "fashion accessory, much like a piece of jewelry or a scarf." The plans were to change the packaging several times a year to coincide with seasonal changes in women's clothing. An internal cigarette company document on another cigarette called Dakota was leaked to the press. The target audience for this product reportedly included "women who attend tractor pulls."

Cigarette companies have saturated women's magazines with advertisements for cigarettes. Of the 20 magazines receiving the greatest amount of cigarette advertising revenue in 1985, eight were women's magazines (*Better Homes and Gardens, Family Circle, Woman's Day, McCall's, Ladies' Home Journal, Redbook, Cosmopolitan,* and *Glamour*). A study conducted in our lab indicates a marked targeting of women over the past 20 years. In this study, we tabulated all advertisements from every issue of two male-oriented magazines (*Golf* and *Forbes*) and two female-oriented magazines (*Vogue* and *Redbook*) from 1965 to 1990. *Golf* and *Forbes* both have a 98 percent male readership; *Vogue* and *Redbook* both have a 90 percent female readership.

We tracked the percentage of cigarette advertisements on a year-to-year basis. In the two magazines for men, the percentage of cigarette advertising rates has stayed stable or dropped. In *Golf* magazine in 1970, 5.8 percent of the total ads were for cigarettes versus 3.5 percent in 1990. In *Forbes*, the percentage of cigarette ads was low—0 percent in 1970 versus 0.1 percent in 1990. In contrast, rates in the two women-oriented magazines have increased markedly. In *Vogue*, rates went from 0.4 percent in 1970 to 2.4 percent in 1990; for *Redbook*, rates went from 1.8 percent in 1970 to 9.3 percent in 1990. This represents an increase in cigarette ads of 500 percent in *Vogue* and 417 percent in *Redbook*. This means that 71 cigarette ads were published in *Vogue* and 92 in *Redbook* in 1990.

A person who reads magazines that accept tobacco advertisements is less likely to read articles in those magazines about the health consequences of smoking. Researchers at the University of Michigan looked at 99 U.S. magazines published during a 25-year period.(15) The men's magazines that accepted cigarette ads were 27 percent less likely to publish negative articles on smoking than magazines that did not accept cigarette ads. In women's magazines, the effect was even stronger. Magazines that accepted cigarette ads were 87 percent less likely to publish negative articles about smoking. A magazine that accepts cigarette ads is less likely to condemn cigarettes in its articles. This is a version of "don't bite the hand that feeds you."

There is strong evidence that cigarette companies not only target children but also you, the female consumer. What else are they promoting?

THE MYTH OF THE LOW TAR/ LOW NICOTINE CIGARETTE

In 1984, more than half of the total cigarette advertising expenditures were for so-called low tar and low nicotine cigarettes. Low tar and nicotine cigarettes account for at least half of the domestic market—and the cigarette companies are seeking to expand this market with a wide proliferation of "light" cigarettes. Marlboro released "Marlboro medium," apparently to entice the hardcore heavy smokers who have not switched to "light" cigarettes.

Cigarette companies know that many smokers are worried about the health consequences of smoking. By smoking a "light" cigarette, the implication is that you reduce the consequences. This is illustrated in an advertisement for True cigarettes. It is in the form of a testimonial from a woman smoker: "Considering all I'd heard, I decided to either quit or smoke True. I smoke True." Assuming this woman heard about the health consequences of smoking, the implication is that smoking True cigarettes is a safe alternative to quitting.

People seem to be responding just as the tobacco companies want them to respond. A 1993 Gallup Poll asked average Americans what "slim" and "ultra-trim" meant to them. The typical person believed that these terms mean the cigarette has fewer harmful ingredients, will help a smoker avoid weight gain, and is designed for women. When smokers were asked what "low tar," "low nicotine," and "lower yield" meant to them, 46 percent of smokers replied "safer."

The truth is that except for ultra low tar/nicotine cigarettes (that is, nicotine levels of less than 0.1 milligram), you do not reduce your exposure to cigarette smoking by using low tar and nicotine cigarettes. There is no such thing as a safe cigarette.

There are two reasons why there are no safe cigarettes. First, no current regulations exist for the use of the word "light" in a cigarette's name, and it is unlikely that such regulations will be forthcoming. "Light" could mean that the cigarette weighs less than a regular brand. Or it could mean a trivial reduction in nicotine content (that is, from 1.2 to 1.1 milligrams).

Second, strong evidence exists that smokers compensate for lower levels of tar and nicotine.(16) Smokers puff lower yield cigarettes more frequently or more intensely than higher yield cigarettes to obtain more nicotine. Have you ever tried these cigarettes? Have you described them as "smoking air"? Have you described them to someone by saying, "You really have to suck on these to get any flavor"? Smokers compensate by inhaling longer, deeper, and more frequently. As a result, there is virtually no relationship between the nicotine content listed on the package and how much nicotine is in your body.

By the way, did you know that the federal government no longer tests cigarettes for tar and nicotine content? We have to rely on the tobacco companies to provide us with this information.

There's one other thing that should make you think twice about smoking a "light" cigarette. Cigarette companies add more additives to their lower-yield cigarettes to enhance their taste. The companies are not required to (and never do) disclose what chemicals or other products they put in the cigarettes to enhance taste. As a result, we have no idea of what additional risks, if any, they pose.

HOW DO THE CIGARETTE COMPANIES GET AWAY WITH THIS?

Since we live in a free society, cigarette companies have used issues of personal choice and freedom to their advantage. Additionally, they spend large amounts of money every year fighting proposed smoking restrictions, and even the adoption of seemingly noncontroversial civic laws (for example, making cigarette vending machines inaccessible to minors). The cigarette lobby in Congress is powerful and tobacco production is a lucrative cash crop, particularly in the South.

One major reason why tobacco companies can get away with not listing additives is that the Food and Drug Administration (FDA) does not regulate tobacco products. Rather, the Federal Trade Commission (FTC), the Alcohol, Tobacco, and Firearms (ATF) Bureau of the Treasury Department; and the Department of Agriculture regulate the growth and sales of these products.

The FDA enforces laws and regulations to protect consumers' health, safety, and pocketbooks. According to the U.S. Department of Health and Human Services, the laws are intended to ensure the consumer that "foods are pure and wholesome to eat, and produced under sanitary conditions; that drugs and devices are safe and effective for their intended uses; that cosmetics are safe and made from appropriate ingredients; and that all labeling and packaging is truthful, informative, and not deceptive." In other words, the FDA requires that all products be safe for human consumption and do what the product claims to do. A product sold as a pain reliever must be safe, and at least two independent studies must document that the product does relieve pain. Neither the FTC nor ATF have such a regulatory process. The FTC enforces the broadcast and advertising laws that pertain to tobacco products while the ATF enforces the taxes on tobacco products.

If the FDA regulated cigarettes, the product would probably be withdrawn from the market because it cannot be proven safe for human consumption and it does not have any positive medicinal or cosmetic purpose. In fact, when R. J. Reynolds was test-marketing an alternative nicotine delivery system (the Smokeless Cigarette), Surgeon General C. Everett Koop argued that since this was a new product for delivering nicotine, the FDA should regulate its use. R. J. Reynolds quietly withdrew its plans to sell the cigarette.

Can you imagine if a label, like the one found on aspirin, were put on cigarettes? Based on the scientific evidence, the label would read something like this:

"Uses: None. Provides temporary relief from the symptoms caused by using this product. When used as directed, this product is lethal."

In 1992, the Environmental Protection Agency (EPA) declared environmental tobacco smoke (secondhand smoke) a carcinogen, which allows companies to continue to enforce smoking restrictions. The mood in this country is decidedly oriented to nonsmoking and getting more so. More and more lawsuits are coming out against the tobacco companies.

However, the tobacco companies are fighting back. The Tobacco Institute occasionally runs an ad that says, "One trillion dollars is too much financial power to ignore." The basic message is that the net worth of all the smokers in this country is one trillion dollars and so, presumably, stop hassling smokers. In Memphis, we have seen a bumper sticker on several cars that reads: "I smoke and I vote." We will undoubtedly see more of this pro-smoking backlash as more legislation protecting nonsmokers is passed. Why? Smoking is big business. In an article in the June 15, 1988 edition of USA Today, industry analyst Roy Burry of Kidder, Peabody is quoted as saying that even if the cigarette companies lose all pending lawsuits against them and pay each plaintiff $10 million, increasing cigarette prices by four cents a pack "would cover the costs forever."

WHAT'S NEXT FROM THE CIGARETTE COMPANIES?

Since the EPA declared secondhand smoke as a carcinogen, there has been increased pressure for creating smoke-free environments. More places, including airports, indoor malls, and entire restaurants, are becoming completely smoke-free. The cigarette companies are fighting these regulations tooth and nail. We are disturbed to see the cigarette companies fueling the controversy by instilling the notion that smokers' rights are being trampled. This is likely to cause a backlash among smokers. Look at any issue of Philip Morris Magazine and you will see multiple examples of lines like this:

> "It's my right to smoke. I don't tell you what to eat, don't tell me whether or not to smoke."

> "I am so sick and tired of these goody-goodies telling me what I can and cannot do."

"First they tell us we can't smoke. What's next? Pretty soon they [whoever "they" are] will be taking away all our rights."

As we pointed out in Chapter 2, nothing will promote self-destructive behavior faster than having people believe they are an oppressed minority and that their rights are being taken away. The tobacco companies are using this tactic to get you as mad as hell. Why are they doing this? Are they championing the cause of the First Amendment and our Bill of Rights? Are they supporting the Constitution (an advertising ploy of Philip Morris)? Of course not. You are their meal ticket. They aren't promoting individual rights, they are encouraging slavery—slavery to the addiction to smoking. Don't buy into it.

We agree with the cigarette companies on one thing: We encourage you to get mad as hell. However, we suggest you get mad at the cigarette companies for promoting this nonsense.

By the way, a common line of a tobacco company representative is something like this: "I choose to smoke. No one forces you to smoke. If you don't want to smoke, don't. But do not restrict my personal freedom to smoke."

If smoking only affected smokers, one would be sympathetic to that argument. However, smoking affects the health of others, including nonsmokers, children, and unborn children. The health threat of secondhand smoke is so serious that the EPA has recommended that people ban smoking in their homes and that communities press for antismoking laws to help reduce illness from secondhand smoke. Smoking also affects us economically; it increases Medicare and health insurance costs, not to mention life, fire, and auto insurance. As a Supreme Court justice once said, "The right to swing your hand ends at my face."

YOU'VE COME A LONG WAY BABY—BUT WHAT DO PEOPLE REALLY THINK ABOUT SMOKERS?

The image that tobacco companies portray in their ads is that woman smokers are glamorous, intelligent, attractive, and thin. What messages do you, as a woman smoker, convey or communicate when you smoke? You might not like what people who don't know you say and think.

Many women don't quit smoking because they are concerned about gaining weight. That concern is based to a large degree on wanting to look attractive to others. This is understandable, all things considered, because we would rather be liked than not liked and viewed as attractive rather than unattractive. According to one study, however, the first impression you as a smoker make is a negative one.

A 1992 study evaluated the impact of smoking on the attractiveness of males and females. The researchers hired actors and actresses and videotaped interviews with them. In one interview, they smoked; in the other, they didn't. Other than smoking, the two interviews were identical. The researchers showed the tapes to hundreds of people—men and women, smokers and nonsmokers. Some people saw the "smoking" tape; others saw the "nonsmoking" tape. The researchers then asked the viewers what they liked and disliked about the people in the tape.

The results were dramatic. On almost every comparison, viewers reacted more positively to nonsmokers than smokers. They viewed the female nonsmokers much more positively than the female smokers—they didn't seem to care if the males were nonsmokers or not. What is interesting is that it did not matter whether the viewer was a male or female, smoker or nonsmoker. In other words, even the smokers watching the tape preferred the nonsmokers. Following is a sample of what smoking did to the image and attractiveness of the women.

- The viewers liked the nonsmoking women more than

the smoking women and rated the nonsmokers as more friendly than the smokers.

- The viewers rated the nonsmoking women as more physically attractive than the smoking women. When the viewers saw the same woman, they rated her as more attractive when she didn't smoke than when she did smoke.

- When the viewers saw the same woman, they rated her as more moral and less promiscuous when she didn't smoke than when she did smoke.

- The viewers saw the nonsmoking women as more physically desirable by men. This is a double whammy for smoking women: they are seen as relatively more promiscuous but less physically desirable.

- Finally, and this isn't too surprising, on just about every measure, when the viewers saw the same woman, they rated her as more physically healthy when she didn't smoke than when she did smoke.

The image conveyed to strangers by nonsmokers is compelling. People stereotype the nonsmoking person as likable, friendly, attractive, moral, desirable, and healthy. It is important to point out that this was a study of first impressions. While first impressions tend to be lasting impressions, once people get to know others better, these impressions break down. So, think of what quitting smoking is likely to do to your image.

I'M MAD AS HELL: WHAT DO I DO NOW?

If you are like most women, you are upset and angry about how tobacco companies have manipulated smokers in general and women and children in particular. You are also likely to be upset and angry about what smoking does to your interpersonal attractiveness. As one woman smoker said:

> "I had no idea what they [the tobacco companies] did to me. I am particularly [expletive deleted] about what people think about me as a smoker. I am angry that people who don't know me judge me just because I smoke, but they do. And I was worried about gaining ten pounds when I quit!"

We propose you channel your anger into something productive. We are not going to propose that cigarettes be outlawed. Making cigarettes illegal would create a huge black market for them and would probably not alter smoking rates significantly. We learned from Prohibition that outlawing alcohol did not affect rates of drinking in this country; in fact, it served to increase alcohol consumption. Large taxes on cigarettes may deter a few people, but people have an uncanny knack for finding enough money to buy cigarettes.

We propose that women smokers fight back by hitting cigarette companies where it hurts most—their pocketbooks. The most effective thing an individual citizen can do against a large company is an economic boycott. We propose that you quit smoking, support smokers who try to quit, and encourage others to do the same. Support stop-smoking programs. Work on local ordinances to ban cigarette advertisements. Work to ban access to vending machines (the most common place where young people illegally purchase cigarettes). Put pressure on local, state, and federal officials to channel more money into antismoking programs and to make it harder for cigarette companies to do business. Don't invest in any stock funds that buy and sell tobacco stocks. Organize and legally picket business establishments that actively promote pro-smoking paraphernalia such as Marlboro Gear. (By the way, did you know that the original Marlboro man died of lung cancer?)

Don't let the bastards take your money any longer.

PART II
A STEP-BY-STEP GUIDE TO QUITTING—AND STAYING QUIT!

4

SHOULD I USE
NICOTINE REPLACEMENT?

By now, you should have all the information you need to start down the road to smoking cessation. You have learned the reasons why people smoke and why it is so difficult to quit. You know that you, as a woman, smoke for different reasons than men, and that specific techniques will help you quit smoking. You have learned how cigarette companies have manipulated you, promising you a positive image when in fact research has shown that smoking communicates a negative one.

At this point, you need to ask yourself whether you are at least contemplating trying to quit smoking. If the answer to that question is no, skim Part II and keep this book for when you are ready to quit. Don't wait too long, though. A smoking-related disease can happen at any time to anyone—you don't want to hear a physician tell you that it's too late. If you are ready, read on and read carefully.

Most women have strong feelings about using the nicotine patch or nicotine gum. Millions of smokers have used one or both of these products. However, there is much confusion and misinformation about what these products are, what they will do for you and, more importantly, what they *won't* do. Many women who come to our clinic ask us about these products and use them. Their comments are enlightening and, in some cases, extremely funny:

Terry: "The only way the patch can help me is if I put it over my mouth."

Diane: "I've been using nicotine gum, but it's so tough to keep those things lit!"

In this chapter, we will first discuss the stop smoking aids that are available on the market. As it turns out, only two have been shown to help people quit smoking: the nicotine patch and nicotine gum.(1) Next, we answer common questions about these products and compare the advantages and disadvantages of each. It may surprise you to learn that just because the patch is "in" right now doesn't necessarily mean that it is the best choice for all women. Finally, if you decide to use the patch or gum along with this program, we will tell you some dos and don'ts about using these products.

It is important to point out that the information in this book in no way replaces your need to discuss this matter with your physician. Only your physician, with your input, can decide whether or not nicotine replacement is for you and what type of replacement is best.

WHICH PRODUCTS REALLY WORK?

In the past, a number of over-the-counter products (products available without a prescription) have been marketed as stop-smoking aids, including Bantron, One Step at a Time Filters, Stop-Easy, IN-TROL, and E-Z Quit. Most studies found that these products were more effective than placebos. So in June 1993, the FDA announced that it was taking them off the market. Since existing supplies can be sold, you may see these in your local drug store for some time. Do not buy any of them, however; they won't help you.

If you are concerned only with post-cessation weight gain, consider the over-the-counter appetite suppressant phenyl-propanolamine (PPA); for example, Stay Trim. In two studies,

PPA significantly reduced post-cessation weight gain.(2) It also appears to positively affect the increased appetite many smokers report following cessation. Although it does not affect any other smoking withdrawal symptoms such as tension or cravings for a cigarette, PPA is non-addictive, which is a potential problem, albeit small, with nicotine gum and probably the patch. If you suffer from weight-related *and* general smoking withdrawal symptoms, consider other alternatives.

But forget about clonidine. Although some studies in the late 1980s suggested that this drug for treating high blood pressure might help people quit smoking and improve withdrawal symptoms, more recent studies have been negative.(3) As a result, clonidine may not be marketed for smoking cessation.

Only two products have been approved by the FDA for the treatment of smoking cessation: nicotine gum, marketed by Marion Merrell Dow, and the nicotine patch, currently marketed by four different companies.

How do these products work? Very simply, actually. The addictive drug in cigarettes is nicotine. Both the patch and gum have nicotine in them, nothing more, nothing less. The patch and gum really differ in only one way—how the nicotine is administered. The nicotine in the patch is called *transdermal*, meaning that it gets absorbed through contact with the skin. The nicotine in nicotine gum is absorbed through the mucosa in your mouth. When you quit smoking, your body starts craving nicotine. The reason both the patch and nicotine gum are called *nicotine replacement therapy* is that they provide a temporary substitute for the nicotine you receive when you smoke. As a result, this replacement of nicotine reduces withdrawal symptoms.(4)

What is the advantage? There are two major reasons we smoke: smoking has strong psychological and pharmacological (or drug) effects. The psychological effects of smoking are as strong, if not stronger, than the drug effects. The idea behind nicotine replacement is that many people are overwhelmed when they try to cope with both the psychological and the pharmacological effects of quitting.

Using some form of nicotine replacement lets you first overcome the psychological aspects of quitting. Once you have confronted these issues, you can gradually be "weaned" from the patch or gum. You should be able to handle the moderate levels of physical withdrawal that you might experience when you go off the patch or gum. Again, much depends on how addicted you are to cigarettes. If you experience minimal withdrawal symptoms, you should be able to handle both simultaneously. If you have moderate to strong withdrawal symptoms, consider dealing with the psychological and the physical symptoms one at a time.

Nicotine gum is currently available in the United States in only a 2-milligram dose. A larger dosage, 4 milligrams, is widely used in Europe. Studies with 4-milligram gum are currently being conducted in the United States and we expect that dosage to be available here in the near future. It wouldn't surprise us to see 2-milligram gum available without a prescription (after all, you can buy cigarettes without a prescription and they are much more dangerous).

Several studies have shown that both the patch and gum, along with a behavioral stop-smoking program, outperform placebo patch or gum alone when either is used with a behavioral stop-smoking program. To date, no large-scale study has directly compared the patch to nicotine gum, but results are comparable across studies. In other words, if you correctly use either products you are more likely to quit than if you don't use the patch or gum; it does not seem to matter which product you use.

When deciding to use a drug adjunct for smoking cessation, we recommend that you consider only the tried and true products; the patch or gum.

COMMON QUESTIONS
ABOUT THE PATCH AND GUM

"How do I know if nicotine replacement is right for me?"

Based on research conducted largely on nicotine gum (the gum has been available in the United States since 1984), people in the United States who are likely to benefit from some form of nicotine replacement are those who have smoked heavily (consistently 15 or more cigarettes per day), have smoked for long periods of time, and who are not only psychologically addicted to cigarettes but physically addicted as well.

How do you know if you have a physical addiction? Ask yourself the following questions, which are based on information in the 1990 *Physician's Desk Reference*.

- Do you prefer higher nicotine cigarettes?

- Do you inhale frequently and deeply?

- Do you usually smoke your first cigarette within 30 minutes of rising?

- Do you find the first cigarette in the morning the hardest to give up?

- Do you smoke more in the morning than the rest of the day?

- Do you find it difficult to refrain from smoking in places where it is forbidden?

- Do you smoke even when you are so ill that you are confined to bed most of the day?

If you answered yes to several of these questions, then nicotine replacement might be right for you.

Additionally, you can use your previous cessation attempts as a guide. Take a close look at when and why you relapsed in previous cessation attempts. Did you typically relapse within a two-week period—the period when withdrawal symptoms are at their worst? Were the first few days "murder?" Did you relapse because you were miserable? Did you constantly crave a cigarette the last few times you quit smoking? If you answer yes to these questions, then consider either the patch or gum.

You may be able to quit without the assistance of the patch or gum if you had minimal or manageable levels of withdrawal symptoms during your last cessation attempt; were able to stop for five, six, or more months; or relapsed for reasons other than a strong craving for a cigarette. We recommend that you read the rest of this chapter, however, to be fully informed about the patch and gum.

It is difficult to predict, from one cessation attempt to another, how severe your withdrawal symptoms might be. Some people who experienced severe withdrawal symptoms during one cessation attempt may have an easier time during the next attempt, and vice versa.

"Shouldn't I be able to quit without using drugs?"

There is a general attitude among people that one should only use drugs when they are really needed. In most cases this is an excellent recommendation and, all other things being equal, it would probably be preferable to quit without nicotine replacement therapy—if for no other reason than the cost of the patch or gum. However, it is much better to use the patch or gum if you wouldn't quit smoking otherwise. If you experience serious withdrawal symptoms, don't refuse the relief you will get with the patch or gum just because you think you should be able to quit without drugs.

In this situation, view withdrawal symptoms as a "pain" you are experiencing, such as with arthritis. If you have knee pain from arthritis, you might go to a doctor to get relief. If the pain is mild, the physician might suggest physical therapy first. However, if the pain persists, she or he may give you medication to help with the pain and reduce swelling. We recommend you approach smoking cessation and withdrawal symptoms the same way. Try to quit smoking without nicotine replacement. If you fail due to withdrawal symptoms such as craving for a cigarette, then talk to your doctor about some form of nicotine replacement. If you already know that you will suffer from serious withdrawal symptoms, you should consider using a two-prong attack: this book as your behavioral program and nicotine replacement in consultation with your physician. It is very important, when using nicotine replacement, that you consult with your physician and follow what she or he recommends.

"Isn't using nicotine replacement just as bad for you as smoking?"

The answer to this question is almost certainly no. There have been no adverse reports (other than some minor side effects) on the short-term use of the patch or gum.(4) When you smoke, you expose your body to over 4,000 different chemicals and particles.(5) Twenty-three of these are confirmed carcinogens and an additional five are suspected carcinogens.(6) Additionally, as we pointed out in Chapter 3, cigarette companies can and do add flavors to the cigarettes and do not have to disclose what these flavors are. They often add sulfur to cigarettes to keep them burning. When you quit smoking, you get rid of all these chemicals. Most important, you get rid of the harmful tars (that occur as a result of the burning of the cigarette), which have been associated with cancer.(7)

When you use the nicotine patch or gum, you eliminate all these health hazards with the exception of nicotine. Moreover, while this is more true of nicotine gum than the patch, your blood levels of nicotine will generally be lower on nicotine replacement.(8) In fact, if you stayed on nicotine replacement for the rest of your life (which is not recommended), you would be safer. Our point is that the negative health consequences of staying on the patch or gum, for the periods recommended by the manufacturer, are minimal or nonexistent.

"Can I get hooked on the patch or gum just like I got hooked on cigarettes? Am I trading one addiction for another?"

For most people, the answer is no. For a small number of smokers, the answer may be yes. The nicotine you get from the patch or gum is probably not as physically addicting as the nicotine from cigarettes.(9) Don't underestimate the power of psychological addiction to cigarettes—you won't have those issues to deal with when you try to get off the patch or gum.

The only real way we can determine if people are getting hooked on nicotine replacement is to see what percentage of people are using nicotine replacement for extended periods beyond what the manufacturer recommends. With nicotine gum, one long-term study suggested that up to 46 percent of users of nicotine gum were regularly using it beyond the recommended four-month period, but this number dropped to 17 percent by the ten-month mark.(10) The study also concluded that gradual reduction of the gum did not lead to withdrawal or increase the probability of relapse.

To date, we are aware of no study with the nicotine patch since the product is still too new. However, because the products both deliver nicotine, we suspect that the risk of long-term abuse for the patch is probably similar to or perhaps lower than that of the gum.

There is some small risk of continued abuse of nicotine replacement. You must weigh this against the probability of not being able to quit otherwise due to intense withdrawal symptoms. We personally believe the fairly low probability of abuse, compared with the health consequences of smoking, makes such replacement products worth the risk.

"Do people relapse after they quit using the patch or nicotine gum?"

Relapses are rare, but they do happen.(11) Typically, people relapse within a short period of time: about half of them occur within a two-week period. So, if you make it two weeks without relapsing you have a better than average chance of making it. Few people relapse after a six-month period.

Studies primarily conducted with nicotine gum show there has been a small but noticeable increase in relapse at the six-month point, when nicotine gum is typically terminated. We suspect that much of this is due to improper "weaning" from the patch or gum. Also, people probably weren't aware that they would experience some withdrawal cravings and weren't prepared to deal with it. Still, the small degree of relapse does not offset the benefit of nicotine replacement for those with severe withdrawal symptoms.(12)

"I've heard that there's more than one type of patch. Which one is right for me?"

Table 1 lists the one company that offers nicotine gum and the four different companies that offer the patch; the table also includes the dosages for each product.

With nicotine gum, you regulate the dose by the number of pieces you chew per day. In contrast, the amount of nicotine you get from the patch is fixed every day; a doctor selects the dosage based on the information you provide. Typically, companies offer three different dosages, 7, 14, or 21 milligrams (plus or minus a few milligrams). Some companies offer a 24-hour patch, while others offer a 16-hour patch.

TABLE 1
AVAILABLE NICOTINE REPLACEMENT THERAPIES

	Manufacturer	Dosage(s)	Length of Treatment
Nicotine gum	Marion Merrell Dow	2 mg 12 pcs/daily	Not to exceed 4 months
Nicotine patch	Marion Merrell Dow	7, 14, 21 mg	1–2 weeks per dose
	Ciba Geigy	7, 14, 21 mg	1–2 weeks per dose
	Lederle	11, 22 mg	1–2 weeks per dose
	Parke Davis	5, 10, 15 mg	1–2 weeks per dose

The highest doses (21 or 22 milligrams) are typically for individuals who smoke often during the day, and who have had the habit for years. Because women metabolize nicotine slower than men, these doses may be a bit high for most women, particularly those with small frames.(13) Consult with your physician before using the high-doses products. The intermediate dosage (10–14 milligrams) is appropriate for many light to moderate female smokers. The lowest dose (7 milligrams) is usually a step-down dose—which you graduate to after using a higher dose for a period of time.

Once you have decided on a dose, you need to choose a 16-hour or 24-hour patch. The 24-hour patch keeps your nicotine at a therapeutic level throughout the day and night. If you crave cigarettes early in the morning or if you smoke during the night, you probably need the 24-hour patch. But if you smoke very little in the morning and do not crave cigarettes then, the 16-hour patch may be right for you.

Provide as much information as possible about your smoking habit to your physician; that way, both of you can decide on the best patch for you.

"Can I cheat and have a cigarette or two when using the patch or nicotine gum?"

Absolutely not! Several deaths have occurred when people wore the patch and smoked. It is unclear why this has happened although nicotine overdose might be the cause. It is also unknown whether these deaths were directly attributable to the patch. While there have been no deaths reported with nicotine gum use and smoking, you risk overdosing on nicotine. If you relapse, discontinue nicotine replacement products. The package inserts for the patch and gum clearly state you should not smoke while using these products.

"Should I use nicotine gum, or the patch, or this program?"

If you decide to use some type of nicotine replacement therapy, you should use the patch or gum *and* this behavioral stop-smoking program.

From the beginning, the manufacturers of these products have recognized that while nicotine replacement helps deal with the physiological aspects of stopping smoking, it does not deal with the psychological aspects. Even the FDA has tied a stop-smoking program to the use of the nicotine gum or patch. The 1990 *Physician's Desk Reference* states that "[Nicotine replacement] is indicated as a temporary aid to the cigarette smoker seeking to give up his or her smoking habit while participating in a behavioral modification program under medical supervision."

Unfortunately, many smokers who use the patch or gum ignore these instructions and, by not using a behavioral program, seriously decrease their odds of quitting. Again, use nicotine replacement products with the techniques and strategies you learn in this book.

NICOTINE GUM VERSUS THE PATCH

While nicotine gum has been available for several years, the patch has only been available for a short while. The popularity of the patch, however, exceeded even the manufacturers' wildest expectations. Many manufacturers ran out of the product right after its release. Since then, the demand for the patch has eased a bit, but it is still exceedingly popular.

While the patch is certainly newer and more popular, it is not necessarily more effective. While definitive studies have yet to be conducted, it appears that the patch is no more effective than nicotine gum in helping you quit smoking.(14) However, there are some distinct advantages and disadvantages to each product. These are listed in Table 2.

TABLE 2
RELATIVE ADVANTAGES AND DISADVANTAGES
OF NICOTINE GUM VERSUS THE PATCH

	Nicotine Gum	*Patch*
Ease of use	Fair	Excellent
Number of daily doses	10–12 is recommended	1
	Not to exceed 30 a day	
Self-dosing	Excellent	Poor
General withdrawal reduction	Good	Excellent
Weight and appetite reduction	Good	Poor
Average cost	$90.00	$120.00

Probably the most significant advantage of the patch is the ease of use. You put the patch on once a day and forget it. In contrast, you have to chew 10–12 pieces of nicotine gum, which is the recommended dose, or up to 30 if you need them, each day. If you can't or don't like to chew gum, the patch is clearly easier to use. The gum is commonly described as a hassle. You have to give it 10–15 chews and then nestle it between your cheek and gum; and you shouldn't use it right after meals and after drinking fluids. Because of this, people tend to chew it incorrectly or not chew it enough. Since the patch is easy to use, people are more likely to use it, like it, and not make mistakes. The only real mistake people make when they use the patch is not moving it around on the body. If you always apply it in the same spot, you are likely to develop skin rashes. Sometimes people who forget to use it one day, put two on the next day. Only put *one* on—never have more than one on at a time.

You can use nicotine gum when you are very tempted to smoke. We know many women ex-smokers who keep a package of nicotine gum in their purse for years after they quit. Use it only when you need it, and pattern nicotine gum use after your normal smoking patterns.

Sara, for example, never smoked in the morning. In fact,

she had her first cigarette in the car after dropping the kids off at school. Because she wasn't allowed to smoke at work, she didn't smoke again until her lunch break. She smoked most of her cigarettes in the evening at home. When she quit smoking, she was able to use nicotine gum exactly at the times she'd reach for a cigarette.

Elizabeth's workplace went smoke-free just about the time she was ready to quit. She was able to use nicotine gum at work, at the same times and places where she used to be able to smoke.

Another major difference between the nicotine patch and gum is their effect on withdrawal symptoms. While definitive studies have yet to be conducted, it appears that the patch is better at reducing craving for a cigarette—which is the symptom that worries smokers most—and other withdrawal symptoms.[15]

Other withdrawal symptoms that are particularly important for women are weight gain and changes in appetite.[16] Most studies find nicotine gum to be effective at reducing post-cessation weight gain and appetite.[17] However, the patch does not reduce post-cessation weight gain. This is a curious but consistent finding. Perhaps the fact that you are doing something with your mouth when you are chewing gum discourages eating. A study from our lab found that the act of chewing nicotine gum (or even placebo gum) significantly increased metabolic rate, which means that you burn calories.

Consider your needs when you consult with your physician about which product to use. If ease and simplicity of use are important to you, choose the patch. If you hate to (or can't) chew gum, or if you have had intense cravings for a cigarette in previous cessation attempts, the patch also appears to be the clear choice. However, if you want to use the product instead of smoking, and the flexibility to self-administer when and how much nicotine you receive, then the gum is the best choice. This is particularly important if your intake pattern varies and you smoke a lot or a little depending on the time of day or if it is a weekday or a weekend. Finally, if you are particularly worried about post-cessation weight gain, consider nicotine gum.

DON'TS WHEN USING THE PATCH OR NICOTINE GUM

If you decide to use some form of nicotine replacement, there are some important do's and don'ts. Some of these are for your personal safety, others improve the product's effectiveness.

General guidelines for using either the patch or gum

- Follow the instructions of your physician, and read the packet insert. We realize that the insert is written in tiny type but it does contain important information about the correct way to use the product. This is particularly important with nicotine gum since there is a right and a wrong way to use it.

- Never take either product without help. You should be involved in a behavioral stop-smoking program, such as this one, when using either the patch or gum.

- *Never* smoke while taking either of these products. It is potentially dangerous, even lethal. The warnings on the package are there for a reason.

- Never exceed the maximum recommended level for the product. This means no more than twelve pieces of 2-milligram nicotine gum a day. Never use more than one patch at a time.

- Never exceed the recommended length of treatment.

- Both nicotine gum and the patch spoil quickly when exposed to air. Wait until you are ready to use the product before removing either from the package.

- Never give your medication to a friend who is trying to quit smoking since you don't know whether that particular product is right for that person.

Specific guidelines for the nicotine patch

- Move the location of the patch from one day to another. Otherwise, you are at risk for developing painful skin rashes.

- If you start feeling "hyper" and have difficulty sleeping, the dose may be too high. Talk to your physician if you start to develop these symptoms. On the other hand, if you experience intense withdrawal when you quit, the dose may be too low.

- One of the more common side effects of the patch is difficulty sleeping and unusually vivid dreams. If these side effects become persistent and problematic, discuss them with your physician.

- It is common to feel a slight "burning" sensation for the first 5–15 minutes after you first put on the patch. This is normal and the burning should go away after about 15 minutes. If it doesn't, discontinue use and contact your physician.

Specific guidelines for nicotine gum

- Despite its name, you don't chew nicotine gum like chewing gum. Read the packet insert carefully. The correct procedure for chewing nicotine gum is to chew it slowly approximately 10–15 times until there is a "peppery" taste or a "tingling" sensation in your mouth. You should then "park" the gum between your cheek and gum until this taste/sensation goes away. Repeat these steps for 20–30 minutes, but park the gum in a different spot each time until you no longer taste or feel these sensations. All of this is discussed in the packet insert.

- Virtually all the nicotine in nicotine gum is absorbed in the mouth. It does you no good if it is swallowed since your body cannot use nicotine that is in your stomach. Most of the side effects of nicotine gum use result from swallowing too much nicotine due to improper chewing (typically, chewing it like you would chewing gum). If you burp or hiccup or develop a stomachache, pay closer attention to how you chew the gum.

- Do not drink coffee or caffeinated beverages for 15 minutes before or while using nicotine gum. These products have a relatively high acid content and nicotine gum needs a non-acid mouth to be most effective.(18)

Now that you have the facts on nicotine replacement, we're ready to discuss *how* to quit smoking for those of you who are ready to quit. As we discussed before, this book can't make you quit smoking. Nothing can make you permanently stop smoking, except dying of a smoking-related disease! *You* must decide to quit smoking. If you are willing to work hard and follow the rules and strategies we give you, you can realize your goal of being a nonsmoker.

5

PREPARING TO QUIT:
THE KEYS TO SUCCESS

We have seen literally thousands of women in our stop-smoking program. Their motivation for attending our program varies dramatically. Here's a sample:

> *Christine:* "I'm in the program because my husband wants me to quit."
>
> *Denise:* "I just want my kids to stop bugging me."
>
> *Andrea:* "I want to quit. Do I have to *do* anything in this program?"
>
> *Mary:* "I need and want to quit. My mom smokes and she has cancer. It's time."

From these women's comments, it is clear that *Mary* will be the most successful. Both *Christine* and *Denise* are quitting smoking for other individuals—one to please a spouse and the other to stop the nagging of her children. *Andrea* will quit as long as she doesn't have to do anything! In contrast, Mary is ready to quit. She is *self*-motivated and feels the need. Additionally, she has been rattled by the development of a smoking-related disease in her mother. But probably the most important thing she said was, "It's time." What this really means is, "I'm ready."

The most important question we can ask you at this point is: "Are you ready to quit smoking?"

This may sound odd to you, particularly since throughout this book we have been trying to convince you how bad smoking is. But quitting smoking is hard work; you need to be ready to put forth the honest and diligent effort you need to be successful. Some marriage experts contend that there may be more than one person who is right for you, and you shouldn't get married until you are ready. Quitting smoking is something like this. There are good and bad times to try to quit smoking. By a "good" versus "bad" time to quit, we mean that the likelihood of success is either likely or quite unlikely.

How do you know if you are ready to quit smoking? Some good research, based on two theories of how people change their health behavior, can help you decide. One theory is called the Health Belief Model;(1) the other is called the Stages of Change theory.(2) This research tells us that you will be able to quit smoking when you are *psychologically ready to quit.*

To find out if you are ready, ask yourself the following questions:

- Do I believe that I could get a smoking-related disease and does this worry me?

- Do I believe that I can make an honest attempt at quitting smoking, with the help of this book?

- Do I believe that the benefits of quitting outweigh the "benefits" of continuing to smoke?

- Do I know someone who has had health problems as a result of his or her smoking?

If you answered yes to most of these questions, you are probably psychologically ready to quit. But being psychologically ready and ready to actually try quitting are two different things. Probably the most telling way to find out if you are ready to take the behavioral plunge is to decide which of the following three stages of change is closest to the way you really feel. What are your feelings about smoking deep down inside? These feelings might not necessarily be what you tell the people around you.

Stage 1: "I am not thinking about quitting smoking at this time"

If you are not thinking about quitting smoking right now, you are known as a *precontemplator*. We now know that people need to think awhile about quitting before they are likely to quit successfully. If you are a precontemplator, we recommend you continue to read this book. However, if you choose to try to quit any time soon, your odds of success are fairly low.

Your first goal should be to think more actively about quitting smoking, read more of the facts about smoking, and think seriously about what it will take to quit. Read and re-read the first part of this book. After feeling more confident about quitting, pick the book back up and give it a try. Do this soon. Don't wait years before you start thinking and acting. As a woman, you may be familiar with the term "biological clock." You have more than one biological clock in your body—you have a clock that ticks down until something goes very wrong as a result of smoking. Unfortunately, we often do not have any warning about when the alarm is going to sound.

Stage 2: "I am seriously thinking about quitting smoking but not ready to make a quit attempt"

If you have been actively thinking about smoking cessation, but are not ready to make a serious quit attempt, you are what is known as a *contemplator*, someone thinking seriously about quitting but not ready to act. What do we mean by a serious quit attempt? We mean a commitment to quit that doesn't have a "but" in the middle of the sentence. For example:

"Sure, I'm ready to quit smoking, *but* the stress at work is killing me."

"Yeah, I'll try to quit, *but* if I gain more than ten pounds, I'm going back to smoking."

"I'll give it a try, *but* I don't know whether I'll make it or not."

As we mentioned before, we have learned as sort of a truism to ignore everything *before* the "but" (which is relatively unimportant) and pay close attention to everything *after* the "but" (which is probably what people really think). Someone ready to make a serious quit attempt says, as Mary did, "It's time."

If you are a contemplator, you are further along than many smokers. You are, in many ways, psychologically ready to quit but not yet behaviorally ready to go through with a serious quit attempt. We recommend you read through the book and then re-read the first section. Read more about the health consequences of smoking. Continue to think about smoking and what it is doing to you. Start thinking about what strategies you will use when you do decide to quit.

Why is it important to work through in your mind what it will be like to quit smoking? Because you are developing reasons to quit smoking. These images (imagining yourself dying of cancer), concerns (worries about your children beginning to smoke), and thoughts ("it *is* worth it to quit smoking") will serve as mental gizmos, things that will help you counteract the inevitable mental gremlins. In the 1984 Steven Spielberg movie *Gremlins*, a young boy receives a cute, furry little creature for Christmas. He names this wonderfully gentle creature Gizmo. However, under the wrong conditions these cute furry little creatures give birth to terrible gremlins, bad creatures that wreak havoc on a local town. The cute little Gizmo helps in its own way to defeat the gremlins. Mental gizmos work in the same way to help counteract mental gremlins.

These positive, friendly, "furry" thoughts will help you in your decision to behaviorally commit to quitting smoking. Once you are ready to commit to quitting, you can use Part II to help you achieve this important goal. Just like the precontemplators, however, don't dawdle too long.

Stage 3: "I am thinking about quitting smoking and I am willing to make a serious attempt to quit within the next 30 days"

If you are ready to make a serious quit attempt in the next 30 days, you are both ready for action and psychologically ready.(3) You are also much more likely to be successful at quitting smoking than people in the other two stages.

I'M READY FOR ACTION—WHAT'S NEXT?

Once you have made the decision to stop smoking, you're ready to begin the program. In this section, we talk about the things you should do to quit successfully.

We firmly believe that quitting cold turkey is a bad idea, particularly for you as a woman. Women are more likely to be successful in a program that teaches skills about coping with temptations to smoke rather than one that stresses heavy and sudden abstinence.(4) Think about it: you have spent years of your life smoking cigarettes—it's pretty unreasonable to think you could *successfully* quit smoking overnight. In other words, for the first week or so, we want you to learn more about your smoking, learn what it takes to quit, and cut down on the number of cigarettes that you smoke per day. Specifically, you will be doing seven things:

1. Quitting with or getting help from a friend.

2. Monitoring your smoking for a week.

3. Finding out why, when, and where you smoke.

4. Cutting down on your smoking.

5. Finding the time and place to quit smoking.

6. Quitting at the beginning of your menstrual cycle.

7. Choosing a quit date.

Quitting with or getting help from a friend

As we mentioned in the Introduction, social support is particularly important for women in their smoking cessation efforts. The male smokers we treat tend to want to quit smoking privately. They don't want anyone to know they are trying to quit smoking until they have completely quit. As *Roger*, a smoker who was really in touch with his feelings, told us:

> "I don't want anyone to know I'm quitting smoking. I don't want anyone to know this is a struggle. Maybe it's a John Wayne type of thing, but I want to quit smoking by myself."

Indeed, men are socialized, for better or worse, to be the strong, silent types. This may work to their disadvantage when trying to quit smoking, since they may not get the support and information they may need to get over the withdrawal symptoms and the urge to smoke. Because self-disclosure and seeking social support are foreign to many men, it isn't too surprising that stop-smoking programs that use buddy systems don't work well with them.

As a woman you probably have been socialized to be nurturing, empathetic, and understanding; you may seek out support and guidance. This works to your benefit when you try to quit smoking, and it is the reason why programs that utilize social support or buddy systems are likely to significantly increase smoking cessation rates among women.(5) Having a partner facilitate a woman's effort to quit is the best single predictor of whether she will stop smoking.(6)

What kind of buddies are helpful? Your best friend or a good friend is a great choice *if* this person is a nonsmoker or (preferably) an ex-smoker. While it is probably best if you can find a woman who truly wants to quit smoking, this isn't as important as having good, strong support. The person doesn't even have to live in the same city. Relatives are fine as long as they will practice good buddy skills. A supportive, nonsmoking spouse or partner is also a good choice.

While the best buddy is one who quits with you, that buddy needs to be as committed to stopping smoking as you are. It's a bad sign if your buddy says (and many will) something like, "Sure, I'll give it a try." Your buddy should read this book and decide if he or she is as motivated as you are to quit smoking. If not, find a different buddy, or find another person you can use if your first buddy isn't as successful at quitting as you are.

Probably the most common question we get asked by women about social support is: "My husband (or partner) smokes. What should I do?"

Some partners are interested in quitting as well. If so, many of the strategies in this book (monitoring, setting a quit date) will also work for your husband or partner. Quitting together, if your partner can be a good buddy for you, makes good sense.

However, many women who ask this question have husbands or partners who are not yet ready to quit. If this is your situation, try to get as much support from your partner as possible. Ideally, your partner should not smoke around you (or smoke very little). If not, negotiate with your partner to not smoke in the same room (or anywhere in close proximity, like in a car). At the very least, have your partner smoke a brand that you don't like.

If your partner smokes, does not want to quit smoking, and won't cooperate with your stop smoking efforts, we have to be honest and tell you that it is going to be hard for you to quit. We believe that some smokers almost wouldn't mind if you relapsed. We don't believe that they are doing this to be mean or cruel, but your stop-smoking efforts serve to remind them they need to quit and haven't. By watching you relapse, they reinforce their belief that quitting smoking is too hard.

Also, it has been our experience that many people with certain values are particularly hard on women's efforts to stop smoking. Some people (often traditional men) may view themselves as tough and strong. It is inconsistent with their world view to see a woman quit smoking when they haven't. How can a woman, who they view as weaker, overcome something that they haven't been able to do? While we don't believe that these people are aware that they are doing this, we believe that it is unlikely that such people will be supportive of your efforts.

Quitting smoking with a nonsupportive spouse or partner is difficult. At the same time, the most common reason for a person to come to our program is that her spouse has successfully quit smoking.

The SALES approach   What kind of support should you give and receive? Fortunately, there has been considerable research on what constitutes a good buddy when you try to quit smoking.(7) Both you and your buddy should get into SALES—and the product you are selling is quitting smoking.

Speak to each other every day

Abstain from complaining

Link together

Empathize, don't sympathize

Solve problems together

First, you should **speak to each other every day.** Frequent, daily contact is important, particularly in the early stages of quitting. These contacts *don't* have to be long and they don't have to be face-to-face. Phone contact is fine. We even know people who have sent electronic mail messages back and forth to each other on their computers. Brief, frequent contact is probably better than one long conversation once a day.

After the two of you quit smoking, you and your buddy should make a formal agreement—that you will talk to each other, no matter when or where you are, before either of you has a cigarette. This strategy of calling a buddy before relapsing is used extensively in 12-step programs like Alcoholics Anonymous, and is probably one of the most effective strategies these programs use.

Next, you and your buddy should **abstain from complaining.** Don't turn your conversations into gripe sessions where each of you complain about what an awful time you are having. It is, of course, fine to talk about your difficulties. But try to focus on problem solving (see below) and don't forget to mention some of the *positive* things about quitting smoking, such as being a good role model for your children, how you will live longer, or how you just went up a flight of stairs without getting out of breath.

Also, it is important to **link together.** That is, a buddy system is only as good as the weakest link. Support your buddy's efforts even if you are having a tough time. Most buddies are helpful, but buddies can also bring each other down, as *Tracy* recently told us:

> "Everything was going well—until Friday. I called Linda [her buddy, who also quit smoking]. She was having a terrible day . . . she wanted a cigarette real bad. While my day had been okay, she suggested that we meet for a drink and a cigarette! While she was kind of kidding, I said, 'Sure!' We met, we drank, and we smoked . . . ."

Don't be a weak link or, as in a game of dominos, things can come tumbling down.

Empathize, don't sympathize with your buddy. Research has shown that a particular kind of support is best with smoking cessation and the buddy system.(8) Women who are trying to quit smoking benefit the most by what is called empathic support. This means listening to each other, offering encouragement, understanding, and problem solving. What is *not* helpful is instrumental support—which means doing things for your partner, such as doing favors or taking her to lunch.

Also, it doesn't help to give sympathy and say, "Oh, the withdrawal symptoms must be awful!" Give encouragement instead and help her solve the problem at hand by saying something like, "Those withdrawal symptoms are tough; let's think about how we can get you through this." Offer sympathy when you can do nothing, or little, about the outcome (for example, consoling someone who has just lost a loved one). Give empathy when you can actively help with the solution (for example, smoking cessation).

Finally, **solve problems together.** Keep your contacts upbeat. Again, don't focus on how terrible each of you feel and how either of you could relapse at any moment! These are verbal, rather than mental gremlins, and they can lead to relapse. Rather, you should view problems as challenges; challenges you can overcome.

Strategies for problem solving   Problem solving basically boils down to a three-step process:

First, define the problem as specifically as you can. Tracy expressed a concern with urges to smoke: "I have terrible cravings for a cigarette." While this is not an uncommon problem in our program, it is not a particularly well-defined problem. We all have cravings for cigarettes when we try to quit smoking. So, Tracy was asked to be a mental detective. Typical questions for her—and for you and your buddy—to ask are: When do you have these urges? When are they better? Worse? Who is around when they are bad? Where are you when you have urges to smoke—where are better places?

These questions helped Tracy define the problem more specifically as: "I have a terrible craving for a cigarette whenever I go out and have a drink with my husband."

Secondly, brainstorm alternatives. Once you have defined the problem, think about alternatives. Come up with as many alternatives as you can. In Tracy's case, some alternatives would include:

- Don't drink, at least for a couple of days.

- Don't go to a bar for a couple of days.

- Ask your husband not to smoke when your are out having a drink. (You can also ask your buddies never to say to you, "have a cigarette," even in jest.)

Lastly, act on the best solution after you have brainstormed all the alternatives. Tracy chose the third alternative, which worked well.

Use these problem-solving steps whenever you are either confronted with a problem situation or your partner expresses difficulties. Consistently adopting a problem-solving approach to quitting smoking will help both you and your buddy.

Monitoring your smoking for a week

As we have mentioned earlier, you smoke automatically and in a variety of situations and places, and you associate smoking with certain emotions, primarily positive ones. Because you have been smoking for many years, you need to *prepare* to quit smoking. The first thing you should do is monitor your cigarette intake for a week without altering your intake. Make up a monitoring booklet that is seven pages long, one for each day of the week. We have included an example of a monitoring booklet below. Note that it is small enough to fit in the cellophane of your cigarette pack. That's where you should keep it.

During your monitoring week, mark down every cigarette right after you have smoked it. Put a "1" next to the time and include the code for what you were doing while you were smoking. For example, if you smoked a cigarette with a cup of coffee at ten in the morning, you would write "1C" next to 10:00 A.M. Keep track of each cigarette you smoke for seven days.

Continue to monitor the number of cigarettes you smoke until you quit. If you are like most smokers, you will view monitoring as a pain. Yet, virtually all the women we have worked with consider it to be one of the most important things that they did to quit.

Monitoring is important for several reasons. First, it raises your awareness of smoking when you write down every cigarette. As *Barb* told us:

> "I rented a video of a movie that I always wanted to see. Two hours later, I looked down at the ashtray that I knew was empty and there were five cigarettes there. I know I smoked them, but I honestly don't remember smoking any of them."

Writing down every cigarette you smoke will make you conscious of smoking. This will begin the process of *you* being in control of your cigarettes, rather than cigarettes being in control of you. By being aware that you are smoking, you have the opportunity to choose whether or not to have that cigarette. You may go ahead and choose to smoke, but it is a conscious, not an automatic, decision. By deciding when to smoke and when not to smoke you are gaining control of your smoking habit.

By writing down every cigarette, you will also learn about your smoking patterns. As we will discuss later in the chapter, you will use this information to plan how you will cut back and quit smoking.

Finally, a week of monitoring serves as a motivation barometer. Did you complete the week's worth of monitoring and

INSTRUCTIONS: Every time you smoke a cigarette, put a "1" in the proper space. This will record the time that you smoked the cigarette. If you smoke more than one cigarette during the time period, record additional "1's."

After each "1", record the activity that you were performing when you smoked the cigarette.

Be sure to record every cigarette and activity! (Even the ones that burn in the ashtray.)

ACTIVITY CODES:

A = WITH ALCOHOL   C = WITH COFFEE
T = WITH TELEVISION   M = AFTER A MEAL
P = WHILE ON THE PHONE   S = WHILE SOCIALIZING
D = WHILE DRIVING   W = WHILE WORKING
N = WHILE DOING NOTHING   R = WHILE RELAXING
O = OTHER

5:00 ___	8:00 ___	11:00 ___	2:00 ___	5:00 ___	8:00 ___	11:00 ___
5:15 ___	8:15 ___	11:15 ___	2:15 ___	5:15 ___	8:15 ___	11:15 ___
5:30 ___	8:30 ___	11:30 ___	2:30 ___	5:30 ___	8:30 ___	11:30 ___
5:45 ___	8:45 ___	11:45 ___	2:45 ___	5:45 ___	8:45 ___	11:45 ___
6:00 ___	9:00 ___	12:00 ___	3:00 ___	6:00 ___	9:00 ___	12:00 ___
6:15 ___	9:15 ___	12:15 ___	3:15 ___	6:15 ___	9:15 ___	12:15 ___
6:30 ___	9:30 ___	12:30 ___	3:30 ___	6:30 ___	9:30 ___	12:30 ___
6:45 ___	9:45 ___	12:45 ___	3:45 ___	6:45 ___	9:45 ___	12:45 ___
7:00 ___	10:00 ___	1:00 ___	4:00 ___	7:00 ___	10:00 ___	1:00 ___
7:15 ___	10:15 ___	1:15 ___	4:15 ___	7:15 ___	10:15 ___	1:15 ___
7:30 ___	10:30 ___	1:30 ___	4:30 ___	7:30 ___	10:30 ___	1:30 ___
7:45 ___	10:45 ___	1:45 ___	4:45 ___	7:45 ___	10:45 ___	1:45 ___
						AFTER 2AM ___

GOAL ___   TOTAL SMOKED ___

Figure 3. Example of a self-monitoring booklet

are you now itching to get going? Was the monitoring a royal pain in the you-know-what? Or did you not even complete a week's worth of monitoring? If you didn't, we recommend that you wait a little longer until you are better prepared to quit smoking. If the monitoring process was too much work for you at this time, the work required to quit smoking will also probably be too hard.

Finding out why, when, and where you smoke

After a week of monitoring, you will discover your smoking habits. You will find out how many cigarettes you smoke per day, and if your intake varies. You might be able to see a difference in how you smoke during the week compared to the weekend, or how you smoke during the day compared to at night. After your week of self-monitoring, look at what you were doing when you smoked. You will be able to figure your high-risk times, which are when you particularly enjoy having a cigarette. You may find, for example, that you light up with coffee in the morning, with a drink in the evening, after meals, or when you are bored, angry, or tired.

Sit down with your monitoring booklet and make two lists. Label one "Times when I smoke." On this list, write down your responses to the following statements:

My most enjoyable cigarette is _____.

The cigarette that would be most difficult for me to give up is _____.

Your responses to each statement will probably be different. For the first statement, think of the cigarette that provides you the most pleasure. For the second, think of the situation or the feeling you have when you feel you must have a cigarette.

Also on your "Times when I smoke" list, write down the situations (talking on the phone), times (in the evening, on the weekends), and feelings (when stressed) when you are most likely to quit.

Label the second list "Times when I don't smoke." *Elaine* comically responded to this request by stating: "I don't smoke when I'm asleep and unconscious! Oh yeah—and on airplanes and in movie theaters."

Actually, if you look carefully at your monitoring booklet, you will see patterns where you don't smoke nearly as much. Many women don't smoke much in the morning or when they are around their children. Write down your responses to the following statements:

The cigarettes that I could give up are _____.

The cigarettes I enjoy the least are _____.

I could smoke less when I _____.

Once you have compiled these lists, you will be ready to enter the next phase of preparing to quit: reducing your dependence on cigarettes.

Cutting down on your smoking

Your next step is to cut down on the number of cigarettes per day you smoke. When we introduce this topic many women ask: "Should I switch to a lower tar and nicotine cigarette?" In the past, brand switching was a popular method for reducing exposure to smoking; we no longer recommend it, however. The main reason, as pointed out in Chapter 3, is that for the most part the low tar/nicotine cigarette is a myth. Cigarette companies aren't forced to regulate either the use of the term "low tar and nicotine"—the cigarette may contain only slightly less nicotine—or the term "light"—it may just weigh less. Also, people compensate with these lower yield cigarettes so that actual blood levels of nicotine are no less than with higher yield cigarettes. Some cigarettes, known as "ultra" low tar/nicotine cigarettes, produce a slight but significant drop in nicotine, but the drop is usually not worth the effort. Also, our smokers typically hate these cigarettes and won't stay on them. They say: "It's like inhaling air: you have to draw too hard to taste anything," and, "My cheeks hurt from sucking so hard."

By the time you quit you will have reduced the number of cigarettes you smoke per day by 50 percent. However, you will be doing this slowly, cutting down 25 percent per week for two weeks. It is important that you continue to monitor your intake in your monitoring booklet so you can evaluate your progress.

There are four reasons why cutting down is important:

1. There is a relationship between number of cigarettes and disease. In contrast to the myth of the "safer" cigarette, research has shown that the more you smoke, the more at risk you are for a smoking-related disease. By cutting down you probably reduce your risk.

2. You also reduce the number and intensity of withdrawal symptoms. Once you get down to 50 percent of your original intake your blood nicotine levels will be lower. When you quit you should be less addicted to smoking. This should reduce your withdrawal symptoms in intensity and number.

3. Cutting down causes you to pay close attention to your smoking. You become more aware and in control of your smoking. As you learn when, where, and with whom you smoke, you will find it easier to eliminate the automatic cigarettes entirely. With each conscious decision about whether or not to smoke you will learn that you are in control of your smoking; smoking is not in control of you. As you will see, the belief that "I cannot control my smoking" is actually a mental gremlin.

4. Smoking becomes more and more of a hassle. After three weeks of monitoring, one week where you find out how much you smoke and two weeks of cutting

down, you may feel, as Mary did, that "smoking is really becoming a pain in the ass."

If this seems like a hassle, good. Smoking was a hassle to learn; you overcame being sick as you smoked more cigarettes and your body fought becoming addicted every step of the way. One reason you continue to smoke is that it is easy to continue. One reason to monitor and cut down your intake is that it gets harder to smoke and easier to quit.

How do I cut down?   Your first step is to calculate your average intake for your week of monitoring. Take into account whether or not this was a typical week of smoking for you. People often smoke less when they monitor. Take your average intake and divide it by two: that's your target goal for the second week. Your goal for the first week will be halfway between your intake right now and your 50 percent reduction goal for week two.

Charlene, for example, smokes an average of 22 cigarettes a day. To get her target goal for week two, she divides the 22 in half and gets 11 cigarettes. To get her target for week one, she figures that 16–17 is halfway between 22 and 11.

Make two monitoring booklets. For the first week's book, write down a number for each cigarette you smoke until you get to your target number. In Charlene's case, for the first week, she wrote for each day, "1, 2, 3 . . . " all the way to 16. For the second week's book, do the same thing until you get to your new target number (in Charlene's case, 11). If you want to cut down a bit more gradually, take a couple of days to go from your current total to your target. Charlene took the first part of her first week to cut down from 22 cigarettes to 16 and then maintained 16 for the rest of the week.

Doing this will give you day-by-day visual feedback as to how close you are to your limit for the day. For example, if your goal is 10 cigarettes per day and by noon you had smoked 8, you know you have some serious controlling to do!

Next, you will pick a set of strategies to achieve these reduction goals. The strategies for reducing the number of cigarettes per day will help you PUT away your cigarettes. Pick the set of strategies that is best for you:

There will be **P**laces you won't smoke

You will make cigarettes **U**n-accessible

You will smoke only at certain **T**imes

There will be places you won't smoke   The first strategy is quite popular: pick situations when you will no longer smoke. For example, you may decide to have only one cigarette at a coffee break rather than two, or to give up smoking in the car, on the phone, or while preparing a meal.

There are two important rules to consider if you use this strategy. First, make sure you come up with enough situations to be able to reach your reduction. For example, say your goal is to reduce seven cigarettes the first week and you decide to not smoke in the car. However, during your week of monitoring, you notice that you smoked only three cigarettes per day in the car. You know that you will have to limit your smoking in other situations to reach your goal.

The other important rule is that you should *not* eliminate situations where you really enjoy cigarettes. Do not give up your favorite cigarette(s). Give up cigarettes that you can afford to give up. Get rid of the easy cigarettes first.

You will make cigarettes Un-accessible   This is, by far, the most popular strategy. Keep your cigarettes in a different place than usual, such as a different room of the house (like the attic or garage), a locked drawer, or the back seat of the car. Some people keep their cigarettes next to them but arrange it so they have to get up for their lighter or matches. This may sound silly and can occasionally lead to amusing stories such as Anne's:

"I wanted to stop smoking in the car so I used the accessibility strategy—I put my cigarettes in the trunk. I knew that if I wanted to have a cigarette, I had to pull over, open the trunk, and get a cigarette. This worked great all week—until yesterday. For some reason, I really wanted a cigarette. I pulled over to the side of the road, got my cigarettes, and closed the trunk. There I am puffing away on the side of the road because my rule is that I don't smoke in the car. I looked around and saw a police car coming up behind me. He wanted to know what the trouble was! When I told him, I didn't think he'd ever stop laughing. I know one thing, I'll never smoke in the car or on the side of the road again!"

Reducing access to cigarettes does three important things. First, although monitoring raises your awareness of smoking, you monitor *after* you smoke. Reducing accessibility increases your awareness *before* you smoke. It makes deciding to smoke a cigarette a conscious, deliberate act. Again, you may choose to go ahead and smoke, but you will be surprised at how many cigarettes you decide *not* to have. To reiterate, limiting access includes anything that puts at least one step between the thought of having a cigarette and lighting up. As *Rebecca* told us:

"I put my cigarettes in the garage way out back. I decided to have a cigarette and said to myself, 'It's pouring rain. Do I really want to go through the hassle of getting the umbrella, walking across the muddy yard, opening the garage, and standing in a chilly, damp garage to smoke a cigarette?' I concluded that this was stupid. Smoking was stupid!"

Another thing this strategy does is buy you time. Most urges to smoke typically last for short periods of time.(9) Because it takes a while to retrieve your cigarettes, it buys you precious time to really decide whether or not you want that cigarette. Again, you may decide to go ahead and smoke it, but you will be pleasantly surprised at how many cigarettes you don't smoke.

Another accessibility strategy is one that we recommend for everyone—have available only enough cigarettes to reach your goal for that day. At the beginning of the day, count out your goal cigarettes. Put those cigarettes in the pack and leave the rest at home. This will give you visual feedback as to how to regulate your intake for the day.

Another way to limit access is to stop buying cigarettes by the carton. It is only a couple of weeks before you stop smoking and the last thing you need around the house is unused packs of cigarettes.

You will smoke only at certain times The general time-based strategy is our least popular strategy, but it is chosen by about 10 percent of our smokers. To use it, take the number of hours you are awake in the day, divide it by your cigarette goal, and allow that many hours between the cigarettes you smoke. Women who like this strategy have a steady intake all day long. They also find this strategy easy to follow. If you have times when you are more or less likely to smoke, this strategy isn't your best choice.

Two other time-based strategies are popular. First, some smokers push back the first (or second) cigarette of the day. Or, instead of having two morning cigarettes, they have just one. By waiting significant amounts of time to smoke your first cigarette you can also begin to practice what it will be like not to smoke at all. Another popular time-based strategy is to wait 5–30 minutes every time you have a craving for a cigarette (the longer the wait, the better). This gives you time to reconsider whether this is a cigarette you really want, particularly when the number of cigarettes you can have per day is decreasing.

Finding the time and place to quit smoking

When you plan to quit smoking, keep your schedule (work and/or home) in mind. Pick a time that would be good to quit. Over the next several weeks, when do you expect stress levels to be high? Are there holidays, parties, projects, or outings planned that you have associated with smoking? If so, don't quit around these times.

Do look for times that may be conducive to quitting. Perhaps the place where you work has gone (or is going) smoke free, you are taking a vacation, or a nonsmoking friend is visiting you from out of town. Take advantage of these times and plan to quit then.

Find four good days in your schedule. Cravings for cigarettes and other withdrawal symptoms are at their peak about the third or fourth day after quitting, so look for blocks of time when the third and fourth days will be particularly good days to assert your will power.

A good place to quit differs from woman to woman. If you have a home environment that supports nonsmoking, plan for the third and fourth day to be on the weekend. Or it may be easier to have the third and fourth day be at work, if the place where you work is smoke free. Some women even quit during long business trips. While these are times that are typically high stress, some women report that they are so busy they don't have time to smoke.

The key is to find a good time and place for *you* to quit smoking. And only you can choose them.

Quitting at the beginning of your menstrual cycle

If you are premenopausal, getting in sync with your menstrual cycle is important for you. It is vital if you are someone who experiences premenstrual discomfort or if you have Premenstrual Syndrome (PMS). As we mentioned in the Introduction, many smoking withdrawal symptoms are similar to or mimic premenstrual discomfort. The seven major withdrawal symptoms are: craving for a cigarette, irritability, anxiety, decreased concentration, restlessness, increased appetite, and increased weight gain. Most of these withdrawal symptoms are also premenstrual symptoms! We know from the research in our lab that even women who continue to smoke their regular amounts crave cigarettes more premenstrually. Amazingly, nonsmoking women have reported cigarette cravings before and during their period.

We have preliminary evidence from our research lab that quitting past the midpoint of your cycle may seriously increase the number and severity of withdrawal symptoms. We have also found that women are less likely to quit smoking when they try to quit during the time following ovulation (typically the midpoint of the cycle) and during their period. These times are known as the luteal and menstrual phases of your cycle and should not be times when you quit smoking.

It is important to time your quit day a couple days after the start of your period. This will give you about 10–14 days before you enter this late luteal phase. Your smoking withdrawal symptoms should be greatly minimized by then and it will be easier for you to quit and stay quit.

Choosing a quit date

Once you have checked your schedule for a good time to quit, choose a quit date. Pick a time, not too far in the future, at the beginning of your menstrual cycle. Picking a quit date helps you prepare yourself for quitting.

Once you have accomplished these seven goals you will be ready, or primed, to quit smoking. Several days before your quit day, read (and re-read) the next two chapters. They provide important information about the quit day, surviving the first couple of days as a nonsmoker, and confronting the mental gremlins that will try to get you to relapse.

6

QUIT DAY AND GETTING THROUGH THE FIRST FEW DAYS

People react to their quit day in different ways and we can generally predict who will succeed and who will have trouble based on their attitudes:

> *Monica:* "This quitting is going to be sheer hell. While I'm really going to try, I don't think I can do it."

> *Eva:* "Quit day can't come quickly enough. I know quitting will be a snap."

> *Pat:* "I'm looking forward to being a nonsmoker. I realize it won't be easy, but I'm pretty sure I can do it."

Monica is at real risk for not making it. She sounds like she isn't ready to quit and predicts the worst (she uses the maximizing gremlin discussed in Chapter 7). She is, in her own way, predicting the outcome of her cessation attempt. By telling us (and herself) that she doesn't think she can do it she sets herself up for failure. Indeed, Monica was unsuccessful at quitting. Later, she succeeded at a time when she was more ready.

Eva is also a source of concern. While it is perfectly acceptable to change your quit day because you aren't ready yet, Eva couldn't wait for the quit day. This is like looking forward to your next dental appointment! It is normal to feel a bit apprehensive about the quit day—being apprehensive shows a realistic expectation that quitting will involve some hard work and a little pain. For some people, stopping smoking is a snap. For most, however, quitting smoking involves real effort. By thinking that quitting will be easy, Eva falls prey to the minimizing gremlin (discussed in Chapter 7) or the "stick your head in the sand" gremlin. While it is normal to emphasize the positive in a situation, believing that stopping smoking will not involve some real effort only sets a person up for failure. By expecting that "quitting will be a snap," Eva became confused and concerned when quitting smoking wasn't as easy as she thought. She almost relapsed as a result.

Pat has more realistic expectations about quitting smoking. She knows that quitting smoking will be hard, but she is ready to quit. Indeed, because she waited until she was psychologically ready, Pat was successful in her quitting attempt.

Quit Day review

As you approach your quit day, let's review your checklist of what you should do beforehand.

1. Have you found a stop-smoking buddy? Do you have support to help you quit?

2. Have you monitored your smoking, at least for a week?

3. Have you cut down the number of cigarettes per day by 50 percent?

4. Does your quit day coincide with the beginning of your period?

5. Have you set a quit date so you can be easy on yourself for the first couple of days?

6. Have you made a decision, one way or the other, to use either the patch or nicotine gum?

7. Most importantly, are you still ready for action? Are you ready to make an honest attempt at quitting smoking?

If you are satisfied with your answers, then proceed. If the answer to many of these questions, particularly question 7, is no, take some time off and read through the first part of the book. A few women smokers get cold feet as they approach their quit day. Many women smokers view cold feet or a smoking relapse after a quit attempt as evidence that they are unable to quit smoking. In fact, the research shows otherwise. Most smokers learn more about why they relapse and what they should and shouldn't do. Indeed, one of the best predictors of whether or not a person succeeds at quitting smoking is the number of times she has tried to quit. The average smoker tries to quit four times before she is successful.(1) It is not a crime to try to quit and not make it. It *is* a crime not to try.

Basic strategies for quitting and getting through the first day

Throughout the rest of this book, all our suggestions and recommendations are based on three simple strategies. These form the basis for every suggestion you will read and use.

Expect the best, but prepare for the worst   As someone who is quitting smoking, we *hope* you won't have a hard time when you quit, but we want you to be prepared if you do. We hope you won't relapse, but we want you to know what to do if you do slip. We also want you to be prepared for a wide range of mental gremlins and some weight gain, and know what to do about them. This way, you will be prepared for the worst possible scenarios.

Prepare for the weak moments   People don't relapse when the craving for a cigarette is low, when they are having a good day, when stress levels are low, and when the people around them aren't smoking. People usually relapse as a result of a combination of factors that make them particularly vulnerable to resuming smoking. When we hear women say things like these, we know they are in trouble:

"I don't think that strategies are all that important."

"Those rules seem stupid."

"I should be able to quit smoking without using these strategies."

"I did exactly what you told me *not* to do." (We have given up counting the number of times women who have relapsed started their story with that statement.)

Use simple rules   Over the past several years, programs for stopping smoking have become more and more complex, to the point where we think people get overloaded with information. When you talk to people who successfully quit smoking, lost weight, or quit drinking excessively on their own, they usually say they used simple rules to help them change their lives. They say things like "I just stopped doing . . . " or "I realized/ decided that . . . " The key is to learn simple rules that will work for you and follow them.

The night before you quit

The night before you quit, go through a quitting ritual. Get rid of ashtrays, cigarettes, lighters, and anything else that you can put away that reminds you of smoking. Most importantly, get rid of *all* your cigarettes (the butts, too). If you have an open pack, smoke the cigarettes or throw the pack away. If you have unused packs, throw them away. They are better in the garbage can than in your lungs. If you feel strongly that throwing them away is wasteful, give them to someone else. Do whatever it takes; just get rid of them.

We have heard of people who left emergency cigarettes around just in case. What purpose could an emergency cigarette have other than for a relapse? Leaving cigarettes around is the worst possible temptation. If it is really that important for you to have an emergency cigarette, go buy one. This commute will give you time to re-evaluate your decision. But having cigarettes in the house or easily accessible is probably one of the biggest determinants of early relapse and a strong indication that this may not be the best time to quit.

Some stop-smoking programs suggest collecting cigarettes and saying good-bye to your "friend," the cigarettes. You may think that you are losing a friend when you quit smoking. As we will discuss in the next chapter, this concept is a mental gremlin. For now, suffice it to say that you *are* losing a part of yourself, a destructive part. We don't encourage people to wave good-bye to their cigarettes. You aren't losing a friend—your friends don't try to kill you.

If you live with someone who smokes, ask your partner to be especially kind to you for the first couple of days. Ask your partner not to smoke at home, or to go outside to smoke. Have your partner smoke a brand you don't like. Ask your partner to keep cigarettes out of sight.

Link up with your buddy the night before you quit. Tell your friends, particularly your smoking friends, that you are going to quit smoking. Tell your friends that under *no* circumstances should they give you a cigarette, even if you ask for one. If you are going to relapse, force yourself to go to the store and buy a cigarette. Again, this will buy you time to re-think your decision to smoke.

QUIT DAY: SUCCEEDING
THROUGH THE FIRST FEW DAYS

The transition from being a smoker to a nonsmoker may be easier on you if you know what to expect and understand why you are feeling the way you do. We will look at those issues below, and then offer you some guidelines that can help you get through the worst of it.

What is the first day like?

When you wake up on your first day as a nonsmoker, you will probably notice how little things have changed. The schedule is the same, the morning coffee still tastes good, and the kids still need to get to school. If you are like most women, you will probably be pleasantly surprised at how easy the first day goes.

Probably the biggest reason why women relapse in the first couple of days is that they are lulled into a false sense of security with an uneventful—or nearly uneventful—first day. This is to be expected, since the worst of the withdrawal symptoms won't start until the second or third day. Women are often unprepared to feel worse on the second or third day. However, take heart, things improve rapidly. On the other hand, we have had some heavy smokers report that they were "in a fog" or "in a dream world" during the first day of cessation. Don't be surprised if either happens to you.

Quitting smoking is like climbing a mountain range. Some people think this requires constant progress and that you move closer and closer to your goal with each step. Other people think that the climb requires some progress, leveling off on a plain, and then more progress. Actually, climbing a mountain range requires progress, leveling off, and then going down the hill to make it to the top of the next mountain.

In general, you will make steady progress. Although at times your progress may appear to level off—you may feel no better on one day compared to the previous day—don't worry, you will see progress again soon. Also, and this is something that catches women unaware, there is an occasional reversal. You are going to have good days and bad days. You may not have a cigarette craving for days and then, whack—one will hit you. There is nothing wrong with you when these things happen. It is part of the natural process of quitting smoking. Expect these little "ravines" on the way to your goal—which is to permanently become a nonsmoker.

What is happening to my body?

Over the first couple of days of quitting your body rids itself of the poisons accumulated as the result of smoking. It gets rid of carbon monoxide, the same deadly gas found in your car exhaust, which is up to 40 times higher in smokers than nonsmokers. It gets rid of tar, which is probably closely related to cancer. (It is called tar because it looks just like the material put on roofs and highways.) It gets rid of more than 4,000 other chemicals (including cyanide) present in your body as a result of smoking. Your body is ridding itself of nicotine, the addicting substance that leads to withdrawal symptoms.

The seven withdrawal symptoms are: craving for a cigarette, irritability, anxiety, decreased concentration, restlessness, increased appetite, and increased weight gain. It is common for women to report these symptoms. Again, they tend to get worse on the second and third day of quitting. That is probably because nicotine is almost completely out of your body by the end of the third day, and that's when your body craves it the most.

Take heart, though, because withdrawal symptoms improve dramatically after the third day. All withdrawal symptoms fall dramatically after the fourth day and continue to drop. If you are like most smokers, your symptoms will be manageable within two weeks of cessation. If you are using nicotine replacement therapy these symptoms are likely to be much less pronounced.

The exceptions to this are hunger and craving for a cigarette. Increased hunger may last for up to six months after cessation. Craving for a cigarette also greatly reduces over time, but may not go away completely for years. However, the overwhelming majority of women smokers report that cigarette cravings become manageable—which means the individual isn't likely to relapse as a result—within two to four weeks of quitting smoking.(2) The key is to hang in there; things will get better very, very soon.

Reinterpret the withdrawal symptoms you experience. Think of these symptoms as the body ridding itself of the harmful chemicals in cigarettes that have accumulated over the years. It took years for all this crud to build up in your body; it's going to take a little while to get rid of it. Because your body is cleansing itself and getting better, reinterpret feeling crummy as a *good* sign. It is like when you are at the tail end of a bad cold and you start coughing up stuff from your lungs. Rather than complaining or worrying that you may be getting worse, you should see this as a good sign—that the cold is breaking up and you are getting rid of the congestion.

Sometimes we meet women who complain that they are coughing more now that they have quit smoking. A common response is: "I cough all the time. I was healthier when I was smoking!"

Most smokers know, on some level, that they really aren't healthier when they are smoking; however, coughing is often used as an excuse to justify a relapse. Actually, your coughing might increase for the first week or so after you quit. When you smoke, your body tries to protect itself as best it can from the harmful effects of smoking. One thing it does is try to protect your lungs by lining them with mucus. (That is also one of many reasons why smokers have shortness of breath.) When you quit, your lungs no longer need this mucus, and one of the ways your body gets rid of it is by coughing. The coughing is temporary; interpret it as your lungs getting better and better.

Some positive things happen to your body when you quit smoking. Keep them in mind:

- Within 24 hours of quitting smoking your risk of death significantly decreases.

- Within 3 days your elevated carbon monoxide levels, which could have been up to 40 times that of a non-smoker, return to normal.

- Within 4–5 days, all nicotine has left your body. The pure physiological part of addiction is very short lived.

- Within a week virtually all the harmful chemicals related to smoking have left your body.

- Within a day of quitting smoking your hair, skin, body, and breath will no longer stink. Wash your clothes and they won't smell like smoke, either.

- Within a week your sense of smell and taste are likely to improve.

- Within a week most smokers, particularly heavy smokers, will find that breathing becomes easier. After a couple of days, walk up a flight of stairs. We're willing to bet that it's easier.

One last point: when you stop, you immediately become a nonsmoking role model for your smoking friends, relatives, and children.

What do I need to think about?

The first couple of days can be tough because you are both breaking the behavioral act of smoking and undergoing nicotine withdrawal. (If you have opted for nicotine replacement therapy the nicotine withdrawal should not be as pronounced.)

Remember all the reasons why you are quitting smoking. Have one particularly vivid image that you can always fall back on to help you through the tough times and combat the mental gremlins. These motivating images do not have to be positive, but they need to be specific. For example, a positive image may be the pride your children will show when you quit smoking. Other motivating images may include thinking of a friend or family member who died of a smoking-related disease, imagining your children smoking, or remembering some foul aspect of smoking (how much you can reek of cigarettes). Many women think of the terrible things that tobacco companies are doing to them—including manipulating them and selling death. Other women, who become angry when they learn how smoking makes them appear, think about that. Others think about Pat Nixon, the wife of former president Richard Nixon, who died of cancer (she smoked heavily for many years).

We find one of the last interviews Sammy Davis, Jr. gave most poignant. He said that he had lived in the fast lane, but he had stopped his promiscuous lifestyle, his excessive drinking, and his drug abuse. The one thing that he didn't stop was smoking—and "it killed me, man."

Get yourself a powerful image for the first couple of days. When women quit smoking they are particularly vulnerable to negative emotions that can lead to relapse. There is a tendency to label *everything* that goes wrong with you a withdrawal symptom. We even know a women who blamed her flat tire on quitting smoking. Tell yourself that smoking a cigarette will not solve any interpersonal problems and that withdrawal symptoms are signs that your body is ridding itself of poison.

What should I be doing?

Cut down on your caffeine intake   On the first day you quit, cut your caffeine intake by about half. Since smoking reduces the effectiveness of caffeine by about 50 percent, when you quit smoking the effects of caffeine double. If you don't cut your caffeine intake, you will start experiencing the symptoms of a caffeine overdose, such as nervousness, shakiness, headaches, and feeling on edge, which are symptoms remarkably similar to smoking withdrawal symptoms. In all likelihood, you will significantly reduce your withdrawal symptoms by reducing your caffeine intake. You will still enjoy all of the effects of caffeine, even if you drink less. We recommend that you either cut down on the number of cups of coffee or drink a half-caffeinated and half-decaffeinated mix. Many people use the latter strategy and never notice a difference.

The Four A's   Your support will help you get through the tough times. Monitoring and reducing your intake of cigarettes, quitting at the beginning of your menstrual cycle, reducing your intake of caffeine, and using nicotine replacement—if you choose—will all reduce your withdrawal symptoms.

Your withdrawal symptoms won't disappear, however: you will still crave cigarettes at times. To combat this, remember to follow the Four A's: Avoid, Alter, Alternatives, and Action.

First, **avoid** high temptation situations. Now that you have monitored yourself, you know where and when you are most likely to smoke. Avoid places and situations that will tempt you. Since so much relapse is associated with alcohol (see Chapter 8), stay out of bars and restaurants that you associate with alcohol—at least for a couple of days. (Moderate alcohol intake is all right in places that you don't associate with smoking, provided that you don't have access to cigarettes.) Some women in our programs counter these suggestions with, "I should be stronger than that" or "I can't go through life avoiding bars and restaurants."

Yes, you will eventually be able to conquer these situations, and be strong. But you wouldn't think about jogging two days after knee surgery. Conquer walking first, then jogging. Conquer quitting smoking in low-risk situations, then work your way to progressively higher risk situations. And no, you can't go through life avoiding high-risk situations. Just avoid them for a couple of days.

You might want to warn people around you when you use this strategy, however. *Amalia* told us the following amusing story:

"A couple of days after I quit, my friends and family started calling me to find out if they had done something to make me mad at them. I didn't tell them that I was avoiding talking on the phone because I used to smoke all the time on the phone!"

Second, **alter** those situations you can't avoid. As we mentioned before, tell people you have quit smoking. If you go out to eat, ask your friends to help you by sitting in the nonsmoking section, just for a day. Alter or change your routine. Because you have associated many things you do with smoking, break up your typical routine. If smoking a cigarette with your coffee in the morning was a cigarette you really enjoyed, try tea instead. Drink your coffee at a different time or place; use a different mug—just for a couple of days. If smoking in the car on the way to work was an important cigarette, take a slightly different way to work. Put potpourri or air freshener in your car to get rid of the smell. The key is to break up the habit. And don't worry—as a nonsmoker, you will still enjoy all the things that you associated with smoking.

Third, use **alternatives.** If you need something to do with your mouth, eat sugarless candies, chew gum, or even gnaw on toothpicks. Robert, one of the authors, must have chewed a couple tree's worth of toothpicks after quitting smoking. If you need something to do with your hand, manipulate something, like a pencil or a small rubber ball. In other words, do whatever it takes to quit smoking.

Finally, get **active.** Take a short walk when you begin to experience the urge to have a cigarette, perform a chore, or take a five-minute break. Reward yourself for quitting by going to pleasurable places where you can't smoke, such as movies, nonsmoking sections of restaurants, and museums. If you are at work, go to the water fountain or do a job that takes you away from your work area. If you are feeling stressed, take a five-minute stress break. As we will discuss in the next chapter, "smoking helps me relax" is a mental gremlin—it is probably that five-minute break to smoke the cigarette that really helps you relax. Urges to smoke generally pass within about 90 seconds, so the key is to be active long enough to let the urge pass. You might want to take up a new hobby or restart an old one that keeps your hands busy and is inconsistent with smoking. Learn to play an instrument or take up needlepoint, crewel, or knitting. Do whatever works for you. As *Elizabeth* told us:

"I never had urges to smoke at work, because where I work is smoke free. My urges came at night, when I had nothing else to do. So I decided that whenever I got an urge to smoke, I would clean a window. Another urge . . . out came the window cleaner and I cleaned another window. I quit smoking . . . and I've got the cleanest windows in town!"

The worst thing you can do when you get an urge to smoke is to do nothing. To paraphrase a philosopher: "The only thing necessary for bad things to happen is to do nothing."

Finally, we encourage you to be nice to yourself for the next couple of weeks. After all, you are doing the single most important thing you can do to lengthen your life and improve its quality. Do some things you have always wanted to do. Take some time off. Spend time with your relatives. Don't be afraid to do some childlike things like going to an amusement park or the zoo. It may be important to stop being childish when we grow up, but we should not stop being childlike.

7

OVERCOMING THE
MENTAL GREMLINS

We now turn our attention to major contributors to early and late relapse: mental gremlins. Remember, mental gremlins are what you are likely to say to yourself when you quit smoking. In this chapter, we will discuss what mental gremlins do to you and your self-esteem and, most importantly, what you can do about them.

In the first chapter we discussed how women tend to internalize emotions and blame themselves when things go wrong. Men tend to focus responsibility on external forces. Indeed, if you look at the research on mental health, depression—which is characterized by negative emotions such as guilt, feelings of sadness, worthlessness, and helplessness—is much more common in women than men. When men hurt psychologically, they are more likely to blame others and act out—by drinking, getting into fights, etc.(1)

We see the same pattern in the stop-smoking program at our prevention center. When people fail to quit smoking in our program, no matter what the reason, men generally blame the center. They say things like, "The program was rotten, the therapist was rotten, and they gave rotten advice." They blame the alcohol they drank when they relapsed and the friend who gave them the cigarettes. They will even cite the fact that the group meeting was held at an hour when it wasn't convenient to park. In short, they will blame everyone and everything but themselves.

From a smoking cessation standpoint, this tendency to place the blame outside of themselves may do more good than harm. Since men don't internalize the failure, they are more likely to attempt quitting again. While their logic is shaky, they remain optimistic about quitting because the failure to quit last time "wasn't my fault."

Women, however, tend to take all the blame for their smoking cessation failures. Even though it may not have been the right time to quit or they were insufficiently prepared for certain relapse situations, the failure is internalized, which leads to negative emotions and mental gremlins like "I'm no good . . . I'm too weak to quit." This lowers morale and makes women less confident that they will quit in their next attempt. This can lead to yet another failed quit attempt and continue the vicious cycle.

It is interesting how two smokers (a typical man and a typical woman) can experience the same thing (smoking relapse) and come to radically different beliefs about why they relapsed. Clearly this reflects a difference in how men and women are socialized.(2) How do you break this cycle of blaming yourself when something goes wrong? The key to understanding how one person may walk away from a relapse relatively unscarred while another is devastated lies in understanding how thoughts, emotion, and behavior are related.

POSITIVE AND NEGATIVE SPIRALS

Contemporary approaches to behavior change acknowledge the close relationship between thoughts, emotions, and behavior.(3) This is illustrated in Figure 3.

For almost 100 years, psychologists and experts in behavior change have tried to study peoples' emotions and feelings directly. After all, that's what hurts—people come to a psychologist because they *feel* awful. The experts have tried to modify emotions in a variety of ways, by having people understand the root causes of their emotions, for example, or by helping them get in touch with deep-seated emotions.

Unfortunately, dealing directly with emotions, without examining thoughts and behavior, is an inefficient way to help people feel better. Emotions are fairly difficult to change directly, but thoughts and behavior, which drive emotions, are much easier to change. If you can make positive changes in your thoughts and behavior you will feel much better about yourself and others—in other words, positive changes in thoughts and behavior will automatically lead to positive changes in emotions.

Note that in the figure, thoughts, emotion, and behavior are all interrelated. Thoughts can affect behavior and vice versa, thoughts can affect emotions and vice versa, and behavior can affect emotions and vice versa.

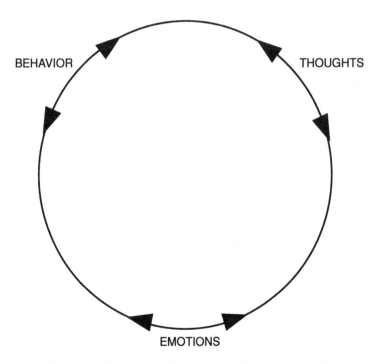

Figure 4. Illustration of positive and negative spirals

This model of how we act and behave drives our everyday life. Have you ever had a thought pop into your mind, such as "I think I'll have some ice cream?" which led to the behavior (eating ice cream), which, in turn, could lead to a positive feeling of satisfaction or a negative feeling like guilt.

Why do we call thoughts, emotions, and behaviors *spirals?* Because they rarely stop. Both positive and negative spirals drive our behavior. Once we understand better how to deal with these spirals, we will be better equipped to turn negative spirals into positive ones.

Let's take the above example and turn it into a positive spiral:

>An idea popped into my head to have ice cream. (thought)
>I had a dish of ice cream. (behavior)
>I feel guilty about eating this ice cream. (emotion)

The person calls up a mental gizmo—a proactive, nondefeating thought:

>Okay, so I broke my diet. It's no big deal—this doesn't mean I am a terrible person. I'll just have to watch what I eat for the next day or two. (thought)

>A couple of days go by.

>I have now watched what I've eaten for the past several days. (behavior)
>I am confident and proud that I can stay on my diet. (emotion)

The positive spiral continues. With such a positive spiral, you can see that this person is likely to be successful at dieting.

Now, let's take the same event and turn it into a negative spiral.

An idea popped into my head to have ice cream. (thought)
    I had a dish of ice cream. (behavior)
    I feel guilty about eating this ice cream. (emotion)

The mental gremlin, which is an automatic thought and is destructive and defeating pops into her head:

Why did I eat that dish of ice cream? I will never lose weight. I have no will power. I might as well give up. (thought)

A couple of days go by.

Well, now I've eaten everything in sight for the past few days (behavior).
    This proves I have no will power. I might as well give up. (thoughts).
    I feel awful. I'm going to go through life being fat, depressed, and alone. (emotion)

The negative spiral will continue. These negative spirals are probably the most important reasons why people, particularly women, fail at their weight-loss attempts. (We will talk more about smoking cessation and weight gain in Chapter 9.) Notice that in both examples the key to a positive versus a negative spiral was whether the person used a mental gizmo (positive) or a mental gremlin (negative). Mental gremlins, which are more common, are intrusive automatic thoughts that pop into our heads. As the above illustration points out, we have many mental gremlins, not just those that are related to smoking. In fact, the best books on self-improvement use the general concept of mental gremlins, although they are called different names by the authors. Mental gremlins usually come into our heads automatically and are self-defeating and self-destructive: "I'm no good at that." Mental gremlins may be idealistic and unrealistic: "I should be strong enough to not have cravings for cigarettes ever again." On the surface, many gremlins appear positive and true, but are merely dressed up to look good. They are, in fact, destructive and false.

In contrast, mental gizmos (positive thoughts) are action-oriented, constructive, and motivating. They are *not* automatic—they are positive statements that you must *learn* to use.

As someone who is quitting smoking, you don't need to learn many gizmos, but you need to call them up often—as frequently as you have a cigarette craving. When we interview ex-smokers about how and why they were successful at quitting and staying quit, it is uncanny how similar their responses are. Virtually all of our ex-smokers report one or two thoughts or images that they kept replaying. Or they report, "The one thing I remembered that the therapist said . . . . " They almost always mention having a mental gizmo which they used in situations where they were likely to relapse. Examples of these include:

"Every time I had a craving, I thought of my poor dad, dying of heart disease. I told myself, 'I will die someday, but not like that.'"

"About one month after I quit, I went out with an old boyfriend who smoked. He kissed me hello and I smelled cigarettes on his breath. What an awful smell! Then I realized that *my* breath used to smell that bad. What an eye-opener!"

"I'll tell you the night that I knew I would never be a smoker again. It started out terrible. After an awful day, I decided at two in the morning to have a cigarette. I threw on some clothes, got in the car, and drove to the supermarket. I got there and it was closed. I headed to an all-night convenience store about five miles down the road. As I was driving, I realized how stupid this was. I remembered that the therapist said that if you feel stupid doing these things that's good, because smoking is stupid. I turned the car around and went home."

"You know what keeps me from smoking? Those cigarette companies and what they're doing to us [women] smokers . . . selling death and trying to manipulate me. I decided not to give them any more of my money."

"I decided I'd never smoke again when my three-year-old daughter, Katie, came up to me one day pretending to puff on a crayon, proud that she was 'smoking, just like Mommy.' I said to myself, 'That's it. It's time to quit.'"

"I always remembered that story the therapist told us about the woman who had multiple chances to quit but was convinced to quit only after she was dying. That's when I realized I had more than one biological clock ticking."

"I'm embarrassed to say what kept me from smoking. It was the stuff the therapist said about smoking causing skin wrinkles, about it aging my face. This may sound vain, but that's what did it for me. Hell, I can lose the weight, but you can't get rid of those skin wrinkles and I can't afford plastic surgery!"

We could go on for pages and discuss other stories, but these illustrate our point. Pick your own gizmo or two. These thoughts may be something you learned in this book—a fact that you didn't know before. Maybe it is one of the case examples that we have written about. Or better yet, maybe it is something that has happened to you (your boss commenting on how "bad" your office smells) or might happen to you (you know that heart disease runs in your family). Maybe you are just plain sick of smoking . . . sick of the money spent, sick of having to leave your office building to smoke, sick of the smelly clothes, or sick of the lies and broken promises of the tobacco companies. You need these gizmos to think about time and time again. They help you remember all the good reasons for not smoking.

Remember to use the gizmos because the gremlins come much easier, are more automatic, and are more destructive. Again, if you recall the Steven Spielberg movie *Gremlins*, there was only one Gizmo, but eventually hundreds of gremlins. And they were everywhere. Unless you are vigilant, you can fall prey to these mental gremlins. You probably have some stored away in your brain that you can think of right now. As we will discuss in the next chapter on preventing relapse, you are most likely to fall victim to gremlins when you are tired or bored or when you have had a bad day. Gremlins might also victimize you during happy, social times—times that are usually associated with alcohol.

Over the years we have compiled a list of the most common gremlins. We're willing to bet that you can see some of your own gremlins below. For many of you, some of these gremlins were precisely what you were thinking when you relapsed. We focus in this chapter on those that are most associated with early relapse, which occurs within two weeks of quitting. This relapse tends to be "fueled" by smoking withdrawal. However, it is important to note that these gremlins can occur at any time and may pop up again later. We also discuss some of the gremlins that are linked to later relapse, to introduce the topics in the next chapter on understanding and preventing relapse.

GREMLINS ASSOCIATED WITH EARLY RELAPSE

Gremlins associated with early relapse usually involve withdrawal symptoms. When you are at the height of nicotine withdrawal and are craving cigarettes, these gremlins have a field day! You are particularly vulnerable because you are adapting psychologically to life without cigarettes and your body is ridding itself of the poisons and craving nicotine.

The two most common gremlins tend to work together. These are the "Joseph McCarthy" gremlin and the "Ms. Ciggy, how I miss you" gremlin.

The "Joseph McCarthy" gremlin

In the 1950s, Senator Joseph McCarthy became convinced that Communists had infiltrated the military, Congress, the White House, the entertainment industry, and every other part of American life. Like Senator McCarthy, this smoking gremlin tries to tell you that everything bad that happens to you is the result of one thing—namely withdrawal symptoms.

To avoid this gremlin, don't interpret everything that happens to you as withdrawal symptoms. That is, most aches and pains are just that, normal aches and pains. If you start feeling bad, ask yourself if you have felt this way before. Maybe what you have is another sinus headache, or perhaps you are just plain tired. Separate and deal with things that are truly withdrawal related versus those irritants that are a part of everyday life.

We don't want to minimize or trivialize the withdrawal symptoms that many smokers experience. However, there is a strong tendency for smokers to become "withdrawal symptoms conscious" and blame everything on stopping smoking. Below are some of the more memorable things people blame on their attempt to quit smoking:

> "My car broke down on the way to work today. I should have never quit smoking!"

> "These withdrawal symptoms will never go away. I'm nauseous in the morning and my period is late." (It turns out that this smoker was pregnant.)

> "My husband just heard that his company is transferring him to another city. This would have never happened if I hadn't quit smoking!"

As you can see, smokers can and will blame just about anything on stopping smoking. Blaming all your problems on smoking withdrawal won't solve your problems—and it is likely to lead to relapse.

A variant of this gremlin is "the withdrawal symptoms are getting worse" gremlin. This is usually due to overinterpreting other aches and pains as withdrawal symptoms. This happens often in the first couple of days of smoking cessation—especially on the second to fourth day when the real withdrawal symptoms hit. Often, women who have had a good first day conclude that they will escape withdrawal and are unprepared for the symptoms they experience on the second, third, and fourth day. There will be good days and bad days. Remember that quitting smoking is like climbing a mountain range—you will eventually get to the top, but it will probably involve going down as well as up.

The "Ms. Ciggy, how I miss you" gremlin

We all have had a long-time friend or relative move to another city. It's interesting what happens. Over time, we tend to remember only the good times we had with this friend and remember less and less of the bad times. This process is called *selective forgetting.* This is normal when a child moves out of the house or even when a relative or loved one dies. Selective forgetting also tends to happen when we quit smoking. We start thinking of all the good times we had with cigarettes; we tend to forget the bad times we have had with this so-called friend. Particularly when we are craving a cigarette or under pressure, we tend to think that smoking will do things that we know it really can't do, like solve our problems and make us happy. Examples of this are:

"I was so much happier when I smoked."

"I never realized how wonderful cigarettes were."

"I may not live as long, but at least I'll be happy!"

You must have heard other smokers make some of these statements. Perhaps you have said them yourself, and believed them. But they are gremlins and they are inaccurate —and we suspect that most smokers know they are wrong as well.

The Joseph McCarthy and Ms. Ciggy gremlins tend to work together. The first starts telling you that everything bad (a bad day at the office, stress, an argument with a friend, a hangnail) is the result of quitting smoking. The other tries to tell you how wonderful smoking was ... even though you know that smoking is really like the poison apple in Snow White: attractive on the outside, deadly on the inside. When both these gremlins are working on you to make you focus on the negative aspects of quitting and the good feelings you expect to experience if you resume smoking, it is easy to relapse.

Defeating gremlins

To defeat gremlins, rely on your mental gizmos. They will replace the defeatist gremlin thoughts with more objective, positive thoughts. Reminding yourself takes effort. Remember that gremlins are automatic—if you do nothing to counteract them, they will sneak into your thoughts and take over. Gizmos are less automatic—you need to make a conscious effort to replace the gremlins with gizmos.

You also need to become a gremlin detective. When these thoughts pop into your mind, stop and think about how objective they are. Would my husband *really* not have gotten a job transfer had I continued to smoke? In the long run, am I *really* going to be happier if I smoke? If you start smoking, you probably will feel better temporarily—you have fed your nicotine addiction. But do cigarettes really hold the key to your spouse's vocation and your happiness? Of course not. That's stupid. And so are cigarettes.

Other gremlins associated with early relapse

There are a few other gremlins that we may encounter at one

time or another. These arise from our insecurities or fears and can be dealt with by rational confrontation.

The "I don't want to become one of those obnoxious ex-smokers" gremlin   We have heard this gremlin repeatedly in the past few years as nonsmokers become increasingly assertive (and yes, sometimes obnoxious) about the health consequences of secondhand smoke. Every smoker has a story about an unfeeling, arrogant, self-righteous ex-smoker who goes around saying: "It's easy . . . just quit!"

Whenever we hear this gremlin, we tell them a story about when Robert (one of the authors), was on a summer internship at a college counseling center. Students who were thinking about transferring to another university in another city would often ask, "Am I going to like the new city?" Robert would ask if the student liked where she currently lived. If the student said yes, Robert told her that she would probably like the new city as well. If the student said no, he told the student that she might have some problems adjusting to the new place.

The point is that a change in your life, like quitting smoking, is not going to change who you are or what is important to you. Are you a considerate, understanding smoker? If the answer is yes, then you are likely to be a considerate, understanding ex-smoker.

The "cigarettes help me relax" gremlin   One of the most common reasons for relapse we hear goes something like this: "I was having a terrible day at work, completely stressed out. I needed cigarettes; they helped me settle down and relax." When Margaret (the other author) quit, she was in the middle of moving. About midday she was exhausted and realized that she had not taken a break. She remembered saying to herself: "Boy, I wish I still smoked so I could take a break." She then realized how stupid and ironic that thought was. Did she have to have smoking as an excuse to relax and take a break?

When you ask smokers to think back to what caused them

to relapse in a previous cessation attempt, a common response is "stress."(4) However, actual stress levels rarely predict relapse.(5) Let's look carefully at this gremlin.

First, physiologically, smoking does not relax the body. The primary addictive ingredient, nicotine, is an amphetamine-like stimulant, which increases heart rate and blood pressure.(6) In other words, smoking revs up your system. In most cases, smoking doesn't help you relax—if anything, physiologically, it does the opposite!

Because many people report that smoking helps them relax, it must be that we have learned to associate smoking with relaxation (remember our discussion in Chapter 1). Why would we learn that smoking helps us relax? Think about what you do when you smoke. You typically take a short break—very often you sit, clear your mind, and think through a problem. While not every cigarette involves a break (for example, smoking on the phone), you often take time out to have one. It's the break from the stress that relaxes you—not the cigarettes!

So, this gremlin is wrong. When you stop smoking, you can and should take a stress break where you sit, clear your mind, and think through a problem for five minutes or so. You will get the same relaxation effect, but *without* the cigarette.

Sometimes people also report that "smoking helps me solve problems." This gremlin is also flat out wrong. Think frankly and objectively about this for a minute—what problem has smoking ever really solved? Have you ever been in the middle of a major negotiation, argument, or crisis, and later said (we jest here): "Boy I'm sure glad I smoke! Having my hair and my clothes stink sure helped me solve that problem! It sure was helpful in there when I started hacking and coughing!"

Cigarettes have never solved a problem; they have never helped with a solution. They are merely associated with stress breaks. Some people chew their fingernails when they are stressed, and people don't advocate this as a stress reduction method! Cigarettes may seem like an immediate solution, but you need to ask yourself (as a gizmo): "How is smoking going to really solve this problem?" Smoking doesn't solve any problems. It only creates problems.

The "B word" gremlin   There are certain words that push our emotional buttons. Men tend to get upset if someone questions things like their virility, their performance on the job, or their driving ability. As the comedian Gallagher says, "Men don't ask directions. They just drive. Eventually, we'll get there." However, women tend to be sensitive about other issues, such as their looks and their weight. And because women have been socialized to be friendly, caring, and sensitive, it is often devastating to be called a "bitch."

We believe that the "B word" gremlin has caused many early relapses among women. The word never even needs to be said—the implication is bad enough. For example:

> "My husband and kids told me that if I was going to be moody and temperamental for the rest of my life, they would rather have me smoke."

> "I was okay until the third day. I was having a bad day anyway and my boss asked me if I was okay. I can't lose my job, so I started smoking again."

The implication that these women were acting like a bitch is subtle, but clearly there. Sometimes the reports of "B word" relapse aren't so subtle. *Lori* recalled:

> "I made it to the second day and was talking to my mom on the phone. She said something that made me mad and I snapped at her. She said, 'We sure have turned a little bitchy since we've quit cigarettes, haven't we?' I hung up the phone in tears and went out and bought cigarettes."

There are several things to address here. First, as we mentioned earlier, people are often miserable for the first several days after they quit. This is *temporary* and you will feel like your old self very soon. Also, don't worry too much what people say to you. Often, their words are well-intentioned but misguided attempts at being supportive or funny. You need to respond to individuals who say things like this. For example, you could say: "I'm sorry; I'm not myself today. I've quit smoking and I'm having a bad day. Please bear with me. I'll be my old self soon."

Not only are you not going to turn into an obnoxious ex-smoker, you are also not going to turn into a bitch. Quitting smoking doesn't transform you into something that you don't want to be. You may not feel well for a couple of days, but it will be worth it. You will be the old you after the worst of the withdrawal symptoms go away, except you will be happier and healthier as a nonsmoker!

The "I was okay until _____ and then that was it" gremlin
This is another common gremlin, which is apparently so powerful that it can undo all a smoker's efforts through one (often minor) hassle or stress. Examples are:

> "Everything was fine until I picked up my three-year-old from day care. He soiled his pants again and I knew that was it. I went straight to the store and bought a pack of cigarettes."

> "It was going great until I came out of the bank and saw I had a parking ticket. For some reason that really affected me. I've been smoking ever since."

Sometimes, though, the life events aren't so minor:

> "I went two weeks without smoking. I really thought I was going to quit this time. Then my mom called. Dad's in the hospital again, this time with a stroke. On my way to the airport, I stopped at the store and bought a pack of cigarettes."

The best way to address this gremlin is to tell you the story of a smoker we talked to a couple of years ago. We were conducting a five-year followup to determine the long-term effects of one of our stop-smoking programs. One of our therapists interviewed *Sally*. The conversation went like this:

Therapist: "So, how have the past few years gone for you?"

Sally: "Not so good. My husband died. So did my mom. My boy—he's nine now—is having a lot of problems at school. They are talking about putting him in a special class. About nine months ago I was laid off from my job and couldn't find work for almost six months. Now the place I'm working is talking about laying off a bunch of people."

Therapist: "I'm so sorry to hear all this. I guess I don't have to ask this next question—how is your smoking going?"

Sally: "I haven't had a cigarette in four and a half years."

Therapist: "Really?"

Sally: "Not one."

Therapist: "How did you do it?"

Sally: "My life has been hell for the last few years. There were so many things that were out of my control. Every time something bad happened, I said to myself, 'While I can't control what's happening, I can control whether or not I smoke.'"

Sally taught us several important lessons. First, notice she used a mental gizmo—"I can control whether or not I smoke." Also, she realized that resuming smoking wouldn't help her through her bad situations. If anything, smoking after something bad happens to you will only make you feel worse, because then you will have to deal with the guilt and negative feelings associated with resuming smoking. Finally, Sally realized that while some things are out of one's immediate control (losing a loved one or a job), smoking is something that you *can* control. By maintaining control of quitting smoking, you can help yourself cope, even with serious negative life events . . . just as Sally did.

The "I feel awful" emotional gremlin   Finally, there are a whole host of emotional gremlins to watch out for. Dr. David Burns, author of *The Feeling Good Handbook,* coined the term *emotional reasoning,* which is one of the most common mental gremlins associated with negative moods. Emotional reasoning is acting from how you feel; for example, "I don't feel like doing this, so I won't." Early relapse is often associated with *negative emotional reasoning,* while later relapse is associated with *positive emotional reasoning.*

While some forms of emotional reasoning are fine, others can be disastrous. Negative emotional reasoning is when gremlins tear down your smoking cessation efforts by telling you how awful smoking cessation is or how awful or weak you are. For example:

"I can't do this. I'm a weak person."

"This just isn't worth it."

"I'm tired all the time. I can't go through life going to bed at 7:30!"

"I'm gaining weight like there's no tomorrow. I'll gain a hundred pounds in a year!"

"It shouldn't be this hard. I knew I couldn't do this."

"I just know I'm not going to make it."

To counteract these gremlins, remind yourself that many of your feelings are due to smoking withdrawal and are temporary. Also, realize that this is a different type of gremlin, an emotional one. Most of the gremlins we talked about earlier are thoughts that pop into our head. However, a lot of these gremlins are emotions. For some reason, we feel that these emotions are in some way more valid than what we think. But emotional gremlins can be just as wrong as thought gremlins.

Most of us at one time or another have felt that we were in love with someone and we later found out we were wrong. At the time, the positive emotions seemed right; we later acknowledged that the feelings were misguided. Often, our most impetuous decisions are based on emotional reasoning and are the ones we most regret later ("My boss pissed me off and I quit. Now, I'm sorry that I did.")

These emotional gremlins are just as wrong. Don't buy into them. They are temporary and will pass. Don't let emotion dictate your decision whether or not to resume smoking—we guarantee you will regret it later.

GREMLINS ASSOCIATED WITH LATE RELAPSE

Gremlins that are associated with later relapse tend to be disguised as "good" reasons to begin smoking again. Once the withdrawal symptoms subside, gremlins will try to convince you that smoking will make a pleasurable situation even more enjoyable. The early gremlins try to convince you how horrible quitting smoking is and how "it isn't worth it." The later gremlins try to convince you how wonderful smoking was and how you would be so much happier if you had a cigarette. Or, these gremlins try to convince you that you wouldn't be lonely or bored if you just lit a cigarette and smoked.

It is not uncommon for women to report that they have relapsed six months, a year, even five years after being continuously off cigarettes. Because of this, we wanted to introduce you to the two most common gremlins associated with later relapse.

The "I feel wonderful" gremlin   This is a simple variation of the emotional reasoning we discussed above. Telling you how wonderful life is with cigarettes is a clear contradiction in terms. However, the gremlins are good at convincing a large number of women smokers. Examples are:

"What will one cigarette hurt?"

"I'm having a wonderful time. I really feel like a cigarette."

"Ah, what the hell!"

"Enjoy life! Have a great time! Who knows what tomorrow might bring?"

We often get caught up in the moment, thinking that smoking will, in some way, add to our pleasure. We have never met a woman who is glad the next morning that she relapsed. People who relapse feel guilt, depression, and helplessness the next morning.

It has been said that cigarette companies, in their ads, are "selling us our own dreams." This gremlin tries to get you to buy into these dreams of happiness, success, attractiveness, and slimness. However, these are simply empty promises. If you buy into these dreams, the result can be a nightmare.

The "I don't need to do _____ anymore" gremlin

Basically, this is a gremlin that tells you that you don't have to use the strategies in this book any longer. But you need to use the strategies, particularly the three rules of relapse that we discuss in the next chapter. We have lost count of the number of times that relapsed smokers have told us: "I know how simple those three rules of relapse are. I thought I didn't need to follow them anymore. They made me feel stupid, so no, I didn't follow them."

You need to be vigilant about following the strategies until you can honestly say, "I am 100 percent convinced that I will never smoke another cigarette in my life." Until then, use the simple rules in Chapter 8.

We want to close this chapter with something to remember and a simple challenge:

There are no good reasons to start smoking again; there are only excuses. If you can find a good reason to smoke, one that isn't a mental gremlin, go ahead and smoke.

Surprised at our challenge? In the years that we have treated thousands of smokers, we have never heard one good, viable reason to smoke. We have heard many excuses and mental gremlins, some common and some unique (one woman told us that she resumed smoking because her nose itched). However, we have never, ever heard one good, rational reason to smoke. We have never heard a story about something that had happened to someone that made us think that it was a good idea for her to resume smoking.

So, if you can find a valid reason to smoke, go ahead and smoke, as you have found something that no one (including the cigarette companies) has yet discovered. Our intent in issuing this challenge is to get you to search your own set of reasons to smoke and realize that they are only gremlins and excuses. Nothing that the gremlins tell you is valid. Stop listening to them.

8

BEFORE I KNEW IT, I HAD A CIGARETTE IN MY MOUTH: UNDERSTANDING AND PREVENTING RELAPSE

This chapter will help you understand why you might relapse and what you can do about it. We will give you the three rules of relapse—*people who follow these rules don't relapse.* We will also teach you how to learn from your previous relapse episodes so that you are better prepared when you are in a situation that puts you at a high risk to resume smoking. We hope you never have to actually use this material, but we will discuss what you should do in case of a full-blown relapse.

We once ran into an old friend who had been trying to quit smoking. She told the following story:

> "I quit smoking for almost four months. I was doing fine. I was feeling great. Then I went to a party. I had a couple of drinks and was really enjoying myself. Before I knew it, I had a cigarette in my mouth. Then, just like that, I had a pack of cigarettes in my purse. I still don't know how I started smoking again."

This chapter is dedicated to her. We have a vision of cigarettes in orbit, waiting for the right time to come to earth and land in ex-smokers' mouths! Or perhaps the cigarette companies have hired a modern-day Terminator, the Relapser, whose job it is to drop packs of cigarettes in the purses of unsuspecting individuals.

Our friend's experience, however, is typical. Men and women who are trying to quit smoking are seldom aware when they enter "the temptation zone." Once the situation presents itself, they exert little or no control, slip, and do nothing to counter the relapse. In this chapter you will learn that you *do* have control over the relapse episode and you *can* do something about it.

This information is important because many smokers who try to quit smoking do relapse, at least temporarily. If you are like most women, you have already tried to quit smoking—a couple of times. The average smoker tries to quit about four times before she actually makes it.(1) You should be able to overcome high-risk situations and successfully deal with them, however, once you are armed with the information in this chapter.

In Chapter 6 we talked about how the process of quitting is like climbing a mountain range—there are temporary setbacks, and you may backslide, but you eventually make it to the top. Smokers tend to have this idealized image of what people do (or should do) when they quit smoking. They tend to think that smoking is like an on and off switch—you either are or you aren't a smoker. One day you wake up and poof—you're a nonsmoker!

Decades of research have taught us that this is not the case. Many smokers have shaky times when they quit. To use the mountain-climbing metaphor, they not only backslide a bit, they head into a ravine. Many people have slips and take a drag on a cigarette or perhaps even smoke a cigarette. It is also fairly common for people to have lapses and smoke three, four, five cigarettes or even a pack. However, it is your response to these little indiscretions that determines whether you go back to nonsmoking or experience a full-blown relapse and return to your old smoking habits. This chapter will help you avoid slips, and respond appropriately if you do slip, so you won't relapse.

Does all this talk about slipping (taking a puff or smoking a cigarette), lapsing (smoking several cigarettes in a row), or relapsing ("damn it, I'm smoking again") mean that we are giving you permission to have a cigarette every now and then? Absolutely not! The best way to stay an ex-smoker is to never have a cigarette again. You are playing with fire in a room full of gasoline if you toy with cigarettes.

One of the best predictors of full-blown relapse is to have a slip or a lapse.(2) That said, it is not all that uncommon for those who have quit to have a slip or a lapse at some point during their life. This chapter will teach you to *not* be typical—and to regain control of your smoking if this happens to you.

WHEN AM I AT RISK FOR RELAPSE?

Research has documented when people are at risk for relapse.(3) Let's look first at why a high-risk situation tends to catch women like you completely off guard.

The first thing to realize about the process of relapse is that the most risky times are not related to withdrawal symptoms. They occur when you least expect them. It is common for someone to report a scenario like this:

> "I wasn't even thinking about smoking. I hadn't had a craving for cigarettes for weeks. Then, I went to a family get-together where there were a lot of smokers. Suddenly, I had this tremendous urge to smoke."

The second thing to realize about the process of relapse is that it is impetuous. It is almost never thought out or even expected. We have never heard of a smoker who has planned his or her relapse. People don't wake up in the morning and say to themselves, "Gee. I think I'll get a little drunk tonight, dance with some smokers, and relapse."

This simply doesn't happen. Rather, smokers are likely to be in one of the high-risk situations described below. Before you know it, one of the mental gremlins associated with relapse pops into your mind and you are faced with a smoking-related crisis. Since relapse is so spur-of-the-moment, the three simple rules we will teach you are designed to buy you time, make relapse an effort, and make you feel a little stupid.

There are basically four situations where people are likely to relapse. Perhaps you can relate to these situations; perhaps you have even previously relapsed in one of them. By knowing where you are likely to relapse you can better anticipate and prepare to confront a craving. You can also use one of the four A's (**avoid** high temptation situations, **alter** those situations you can't avoid, get **active,** and use **alternatives**) we discussed in Chapter 6. Since so much of relapse is unplanned and impetuous, we firmly believe that anticipating these high-risk situations will go a long way in helping you successfully cope with any cravings.

The four major situations that cause relapse

The situations in which relapse usually occurs are framed by your emotions and state of mind.

Emotional upsets   The first predictable high-risk situation is an emotional upset, which can be as major as a loved one passing away or as minor as a parking ticket. Maybe the boss yells at you, or one of the kids gets in a fight at school.

While the mental gremlins will try to tell you otherwise, we don't know any emotional or stressful situation that is helped by smoking. Smoking may bring short-term (*very* short-term) psychological relief, but it *never* fixes the problem. Additionally, the guilt, remorse, and feelings of failure over relapsing make people feel much worse in the long run. How can smoking help when you have just gotten a parking ticket? The dialogue between *Emily* and one of our therapists makes this clear.

> *Emily:* "Things were terrible at work. I borrowed some cigarettes and smoked them. Then I bought a pack."
>
> *Therapist:* "How did having a cigarette make you feel?"
>
> *Emily:* "At the time, great."
>
> *Therapist:* "As great as you thought it would feel?"
>
> *Emily:* "No."
>
> *Therapist:* "How did you feel later?"
>
> *Emily:* "Awful (long pause); just awful!"

There are several things you can do in these situations. For example, tell yourself that smoking will not make the situation any better and will probably make it worse. Tell yourself you may not be in control of what is upsetting you, but you *are* in control of whether or not you smoke. Also, think about our friend in the last chapter who did not relapse despite having several tragic things happen to her. In many ways, not smoking can help you cope. We have had people tell us things like:

> "Things at work are bad; there are lots of layoffs. I was spared this time, but maybe not next time. I was a bundle of nerves for almost a month. However, one of the things that kept me going is that I didn't smoke. I'm really proud of that."

Additionally, focus on the problem at hand. Don't focus on something that won't help the problem (whether or not you should smoke). Problem solve or come up with ways of coping with the situation. Or find a more positive way to indulge yourself a bit—for example, buy something you want, or engage in an enjoyable activity. Sometimes just the thought of having to go through the whole process of smoking cessation again is enough! As one smoker told us:

> "You don't know how close I came to relapse. I was on the way to the store to buy them. Then I started to think about all the effort I had put into stopping smoking and I realized that I didn't want to go through all that work again. I have more important things to do than invest all this energy in quitting smoking again!"

Happy times   Relapses can also occur during unusually happy times, such as reunions of old friends (particularly smokers), holiday get-togethers, and most social situations where alcohol is available.(4) The general rule of thumb is that you need to be vigilant during times that are unusually happy *and* sad. Fortunately, these happy situations are generally more predictable than negative situations. (It's hard to predict when you might get a flat tire.) These happy times are particularly problematic when you are socializing with other smokers. For example, *Amy* told us: "I was at a Fourth of July party. It was a great barbecue. Everyone was smoking. I was enjoying myself so much I said, 'What the hell?'" It isn't difficult to pick out the mental gremlin in this example.

You can deal with these happy situations exactly the way you confront negative ones. Because happy events are fairly predictable, anticipate them, prepare for them, and rehearse how you are going to deal with them. Use the four A's. While we don't advocate that you avoid such situations, you may want to plan on altering the situation by informing your friends, at an appropriate time, that you have quit smoking. Trying to keep your hands or your mouth occupied (using alternatives) may also help.

Activities in the evening with alcohol   The third, and perhaps most common, relapse situation is the evening activity where alcohol is present.(5) Perhaps you or someone you know has relapsed in a similar situation. Evening activities with alcohol are dangerous combinations from a smoking relapse point of view; we may have had a long, perhaps stressful day, and we may be very tired. When we are tired, our judgment isn't as good as when we are awake and refreshed. Combine this with alcohol, which reduces inhibitions and impairs judgment, and it is not too surprising that people relapse.

You can often anticipate these situations, prepare for them, and rehearse in your mind how you are going to deal with them. However, with such a dangerous combination it's usually not enough just to do this. As Emily told us:

"I had it all planned out. I knew I would have something to drink, so I was going to tell my friends I had quit smoking. I practiced my mental gizmos. I kept telling myself to watch out for the mental gremlins. Well, while I only had a couple of drinks, I must not have realized how tired I was. The alcohol hit me like a ton of bricks. You know, I don't even remember who gave me the first cigarette. Before I knew it I was at the damned cigarette machine!"

During the first couple of weeks after smoking cessation, when you are particularly vulnerable to relapse, it is probably best to avoid these situations. However, in the long run this is impractical. You don't want to miss out on socializing. So use another "A": alter the situation. Tell your friends you quit smoking. Note, though, that telling her friends wasn't enough for Emily. We recommend that you limit your alcohol intake, at least for a while. Volunteer to be the designated driver.

This doesn't mean that if you drink, you need to become a teetotaler. You can certainly drink and have a good time. However, space out your drinks, alternate between alcoholic and non-alcoholic drinks, or limit yourself to a certain number of drinks. Keep in mind that alcohol is likely to hit you harder if you are particularly tired or drinking on an empty stomach. If possible, take a short rest before you go out. Eat something before you drink. Because sparkling wine and champagnes hit you harder than regular wine (the fizz in the champagne helps your body absorb more of the alcohol), drink wine instead. Or drink beverages that are less intoxicating, such as beer or wine coolers. You could also order a mixed drink like a rum and Coke, and ask for a large glass that has more Coke in it.

It is important to emphasize that *nothing is more closely linked to long-term smoking relapse than alcohol.*(6) Be on guard when you are drinking alcohol. *Always* follow the three rules of relapse (see next section).

Times of boredom   Boredom can also bring on a relapse. This can happen when the workplace does not restrict smoking and the job is repetitive and dull. Talking on the phone all day or traveling distances in a car alone can also get to you. Relapse from boredom is also somewhat common when women live alone (or their husbands/partners work or are gone in the evening). As *Elizabeth* told us: "After the kids are in bed, there's just nothing to do. There's nothing to watch on television. Smoking, at least, is something to do."

There are many things to do instead of engaging in an activity that is likely to kill you! The key here is alternatives. Have something that you can do with your hands and/or mouth when you are doing boring, repetitive, or menial tasks. Bring along a book, a crossword puzzle, or magazines. If you travel long distances in a car alone, check out some books on tape from the local library and play them on the car's tape deck or a tape player you bring along. Keep yourself busy at home. As we have mentioned before, stay active. Take up a new hobby, do something different. You may not like the first thing you try, but keep trying.

This covers the majority of relapse situations. However, relapse situations tend to be highly individualized. We will discuss how to analyze your own previous relapse situations later in this chapter.

THE THREE RULES OF
RELAPSE—FOLLOW THESE!

If you use nothing else from this chapter, use these rules. We do not know anyone who has closely followed these rules and has permanently gone back to smoking. In contrast, virtually everyone we know who went back to smoking broke at least one of these three rules. As *Deena* told us:

> "I memorized all three rules. I have them written down and carry them in my purse. But, you know, I'd been really good—I hadn't had a cigarette in almost six months—and I decided I didn't have to follow these rules anymore. To prove it to myself, I threw away the little card with the three rules. A week later, I broke one of the rules and I'm smoking again."

We have had people ask us: "Wait a minute. Are these three rules of *relapse* or the three rules for *preventing* relapse?"

Our answer is yes—to both. Follow these rules and they will help you *prevent* relapse. However, if you are bound and determined to relapse in a particular situation, if you are, at any moment, convinced that you want, need, or have to have a cigarette, then you need to follow these rules as well.

You may have noticed that we have avoided the word "must" in this book. We don't use terms such as "you must follow" or "you must do." This is because smoking, smoking cessation, and relapse are so personal and individualized. But we need to say "must" now. These rules are so important that we are compelled to tell you that you must follow them. The three rules of relapse are:

1. Never smoke a cigarette that is given to you.

2. Never buy cigarettes in the place where you are about to relapse.

3. After buying a pack of cigarettes and smoking a cigarette, throw the rest of the pack away.

What is so important about these rules and what are the
reasons for following them? The key is to limit easy access to a
cigarette as a result of an impetuous desire to smoke. The
central goal is to allow time to pass from the point you decide
to have a cigarette until the time you actually light up. The
second rule removes you from the situation you are about to
relapse in, at least for a while. Many times, smokers will tell us
that they don't remember why they smoked a cigarette or why
they relapsed in that situation. Many relapses are situational—
that is, we tend to get caught up in the sights, sounds, and even
smells (for example, cigarette smoke) of the situation. These
rules give you a chance to wake up before you take a puff.
     Let's go through the rules and explain each one in more
detail.

Never smoke a cigarette that is given to you   Do not bum
a cigarette from a friend or stranger. You must *buy* the cigarettes that you plan to relapse with.
     If you talk to large numbers of smokers and ask them how
they got their first cigarette following a long period of smoking
cessation, surprisingly few of them report that they bought them.
     The most common response is they asked for one from
another smoker or another smoker offered one to them. This
reinforces the spur-of-the-moment nature of smoking relapse. An
urge suddenly comes over you and you are attacked with a
gremlin that says something like "Ah, what the hell!" But you
don't have any cigarettes (we assume that you have followed
our previous recommendation to get rid of all your cigarettes).
Your gremlin wants immediate satisfaction. The quickest, easi-
est way to get this immediate gratification is to bum a cigarette
from a friend or a stranger. After all, you only want one. As
Bonnie told us:

"I thought I didn't need to follow the first rule. I only wanted one! It surprised me how easy it was to get a cigarette. That cigarette tasted awful. But the next one tasted better...."

Most women will tell you in these situations that they didn't want to resume smoking. After all, Bonnie just wanted one. Unfortunately, one often leads to two, which leads to another one, and, well, you can fill in the rest. And when you think about it, bumming a cigarette is kind of a weird notion. If you are on a diet and want a snack, you aren't likely to pick some food off the plate of a perfect stranger! Or, if you are at a party and you are thirsty, you don't ask someone for a sip of his or her drink. In both of these situations, you would go and get your own food or drink.

So follow the rule. If having a cigarette is really that important to you, take the time to go out and get the cigarettes yourself. Give yourself time to think about this decision to make sure it is what you really want. We're willing to bet that it *isn't* what you really want to do. Consider the case of *Terry*, who followed the rule:

" . . . at that moment, I wanted a cigarette. God, I wanted a cigarette. I was about to pick up my friend's pack and take one when I remembered the first rule. So I excused myself. As soon as I walked out of the bar [she also followed the second rule] and the fresh air hit me, I knew I didn't really want a cigarette. I went back in the bar, finished my drink, and went home. I tell you, I'll never forget that moment. I was really proud of myself for that. It wasn't easy, but I did it."

So, follow Rule 1. Remember from the last chapter that one of the gremlins is something like: "These rules are stupid. You don't have to follow them." No matter what the gremlins tell you in this situation, it is important to follow this rule.

Never buy cigarettes in the place where you are about to relapse   You must leave wherever you are and buy them somewhere else. You must wait ten minutes before buying your cigarettes.

Many places where people relapse (restaurants, bars, or other public places) have cigarette vending machines. If you are about to relapse in a place like this, you must leave and buy the cigarettes somewhere else. You need to walk or drive somewhere that sells cigarettes. Allow at least ten minutes to pass before you purchase cigarettes.

This rule does several things. First, it removes you from the situation that you are about to relapse in. It removes all the cues to smoke that are affecting you—the sights, the sounds, and the "heat of the moment," if you will. Second, as we stated earlier, it buys you something very important—time. It gives you time to evaluate, and re-evaluate, what you are about to do. We recommend that at least ten minutes pass in case there is a convenience store right next door or nearby. Spend that ten minutes by yourself and evaluate your decision to smoke. Think about the short-term benefits of having a cigarette (one that is likely to taste very bad) versus the risk of becoming a smoker again.

Finally, this process will make you feel a little silly. If so, that's not so bad. As *Shirley* told us:

> "There I was, in my nightgown [she had decided to relapse at home], it's the middle of the night, and this silly urge to smoke made me get in my car and drive to a convenience store. I got to the driveway of the store before I turned back. At least I didn't smoke. At the time, though, I felt stupid . . . really stupid!"

After buying a pack of cigarettes and smoking a cigarette, throw the rest of the pack away   Do not smoke the cigarette in the place where you decided to relapse. If you want another cigarette, fine. Buy another pack, smoke one, and throw *that* pack away.

A few people think the part of this rule about throwing the pack away is extreme. However, the cigarettes are better in the garbage than in your lungs. Also, it's better to buy a pack for one cigarette than to start smoking again and spend that or more every day. Besides, cigarettes are poison; they *belong* in the garbage!

Let's discuss the rationale for each part of this rule. First, women in these relapse situations almost never say that they want to smoke a pack of cigarettes, they want "just one." If you are like most women smokers, when you relapsed you probably never intended to have any more than one (or a few) cigarettes. So, people buy a pack of cigarettes with the *intention* of smoking only one. After smoking a cigarette, you suddenly are staring at 19 (or more) cigarettes. You are now in violation of one of the key rules for stopping smoking—getting rid of all your cigarettes.

After staring at these cigarettes or taking them home, a mental gremlin pops into your head: "I've got these cigarettes. It would be a shame if they went to waste. I'll just finish the pack." By the time you finish the pack, you've concluded you're a smoker again and you go back to your old smoking patterns.

This last rule is also intended to illustrate to you how silly smoking is. While it is rare for people to get this far along in the rules, *Julie* did:

> "Here I am. It's the middle of the night. I've left a wonderful party. I'm outside a gas station smoking a $2.50 cigarette. You know what? The cigarette tasted awful. It wasn't at all what I expected. The clerk must have thought I was nuts; he saw me throw the pack away. At that moment, maybe I was. I didn't want to spend another $2.50 for another cigarette that was going to taste awful, so I went back to the party and enjoyed myself."

So, follow all three rules and follow them word for word. Copy them down, keep them with you, and refer to them when you need to. We have never met a woman who followed all three rules and still relapsed. We are willing to bet that these rules will save you from relapsing in those impetuous, hard-to-predict situations.

BECOME A MENTAL DETECTIVE

In our program we help each woman develop a personal relapse plan right after she quits smoking. If you recall, a common recommendation for avoiding relapse is anticipating high relapse situations and planning coping strategies for dealing with them. Over the years we have found that if we ask three general questions, people can come up with their *own* relapse plan. As we mentioned earlier, after you have gotten over the worst of the withdrawal symptoms, any relapse is likely to involve high-risk situations and mental gremlins. We recommend that you sit down with a pencil and a couple of sheets of paper and come up with your own personal relapse plan. You should answer, in as much detail as possible, the following questions:

1. What situations are you likely to relapse in? What are the places, times, and moods that are "high risk" for you?

2. What specifically do you plan to do in these situations to avoid relapse? How can people help you? How will you alter the situation so you won't smoke?

3. What are some of the mental gremlins that you are likely to experience in these relapse situations? What mental gizmos can you use to counteract these situations?

We recommend that you review your answers whenever you think a high-risk situation will occur. The more you can anticipate and plan for high-risk situations, the better prepared you will be to cope with them.

WHAT TO DO IF YOU HAVE A
FULL-BLOWN RELAPSE

Whenever we discuss this issue in our groups, someone inevitably asks: "Why are you telling us what to do if we completely relapse if you don't expect us to? Don't you have faith in us? Don't you believe in your program?"

Yes, we have faith in you. We also believe in our program. However, we are also acutely aware of the research that shows that many women relapse after a cessation attempt. We believe that you can significantly increase your chances of quitting successfully by using the techniques in this book. In interviewing women who have gone back to smoking, we have lost count of the number of times we have heard: "I did exactly what you said not to do" or "I didn't do what you told me to do."

We also feel you need to be aware of relapse prevention strategies so that you have *more* information than you need to quit smoking and stay quit. Also, it is always best, as we have said earlier, to plan for the worst and hope for the best. We certainly hope you won't relapse, but you will be prepared if you do. You don't expect to have a house fire, but you are wise to have smoke detectors and a fire extinguisher just the same.

Let's take the case of *Emma*, who was able to quit smoking for almost three weeks. At a family function, she had a sudden craving for a cigarette. Her sister smoked the same cigarettes as Emma, and instead of following the three rules of relapse, Emma smoked one of her sister's cigarettes. And smoked another. And another. Before long, Emma went and bought a pack of cigarettes and smoked most of those. She woke up the next morning and said to herself: "Oh no. I've smoked more than half a pack of cigarettes."

Emma is like most women smokers who relapse. What do you think she does to regain control of her smoking? Mind you, she has had about 14 cigarettes. She knows she did exactly what she didn't want to do. She knows everything about quitting smoking that you now know. What do you suppose Emma does?

Nothing.

That's right. Nothing.

The vast majority of women do not even *attempt* to stop smoking again.(7) They go "belly up," so to speak. Despite all the knowledge and their hard work at stopping smoking, most people do absolutely nothing to try to regain control of smoking—at a time when they are likely to be successful. That is, they are likely to be successful because their nicotine levels are very low and they haven't re-established all the behavioral patterns associated with smoking.

Why don't people do anything? Well, they fall victim to a mental gremlin that is so crucial to relapse that researchers have given a special name to it—the *abstinence violation effect*.(8) Emma violated her vow of abstinence or smoking cessation. This releases a whole set of mental gremlins that make her conclude that complete relapse is inevitable:

"I knew I couldn't do it. What a weak person I am!"

"That's it, I've blown it."

"I've got an addictive personality and I'm addicted to cigarettes."

"I like cigarettes too much; I was a fool to try to quit."

"I'll quit again someday; now isn't a good time with my stress and all."

"That's it. I'm a smoker again" (the most common gremlin).

These mental gremlins are no more valid than any of the others we have talked about. As we have said before—we have yet to hear of one good, legitimate reason to smoke—only excuses. It would be a shame for Emma to begin to smoke again just because she had a few cigarettes, or even more than a few. Even cigarette companies—and we know how honest and trustworthy they are—have publicly stated that they do not want people to start smoking. They argue that all their advertising is merely to get current smokers to switch to their brand, not for nonsmokers or ex-smokers to begin to smoke.(9) If the companies that are making billions of dollars selling death are telling people not to start smoking, why should Emma . . . or you?

Emma fell victim to this set of mental gremlins and concluded that there was nothing she could do—she had blown it and was "destined" to go back to smoking. This is simply not true. Emma is not a smoker—she's an ex-smoker who has just had a couple of cigarettes. As we mentioned above, the levels of nicotine in her body are still very low. Also, she has not re-established all her old behavioral habits that accompany smoking.

So, Emma's first reaction to a full-blown smoking relapse is to do nothing. The next thing she did, and this is also common, was to tell no one. She even hid the fact that she was smoking for over two weeks. She was embarrassed, even ashamed, that she had fallen off the wagon. People like Emma often hide their smoking from the very people who could be helping her—her spouse, friends, loved ones, and co-workers. She didn't tell them when she needed them the most!

So, what are the strategies that Emma should have used . . . the ones that you should use if you happen to find yourself in this situation? First, and most importantly, do not fall victim to the gremlins that tell you to do nothing when you relapse. You need to act right away. Second, enlist the aid of others. Contact your buddies. Talk to them about strategies you have learned that may help you control your smoking again. Do *not* keep your relapse a secret—the quicker you get active and get support, the easier it will be to regain your ex-smoking status.

Next, use mental gizmos to fight the gremlins that are telling you to completely relapse. Remind yourself of why you quit. Come up with thoughts and images that may help. Re-read the first couple of chapters of this book to help you come up with new gizmos.

Set another quit date—right away. This is very important, as it is a sign of your commitment to quitting smoking. The earlier the better, unless you are approaching the premenstrual phase of your cycle. Then wait until your period is almost over.

Re-read the sections of this book on how to quit smoking. Re-implement the strategies that you learned when you quit. Use this relapse as a learning experience. As Emma said to us: "Now I know what *not* to do the next time."

Finally, and above all, don't give yourself a hard time. Don't dwell on the relapse. Stay action-oriented. If you dwell on this setback, the mental gremlins will multiply. Remember, the important thing is not that you lapsed but how you *handle* the lapse. To paraphrase what we have said before, it's not a crime that you relapsed from smoking. The crime is doing nothing in response.

9

BUT I DON'T WANT
TO GAIN WEIGHT!

In many ways, this is the most important chapter, so we saved it for last. Fear of weight gain following cessation is much more common in women than men; in fact, it is probably the single biggest difference between why women and men smoke.(1) Adolescent girls are much more likely to report that they are smoking for the weight-control "benefits".(2) Women are much more likely to report weight gain as a reason for relapsing following a smoking cessation attempt.(3) People who do not plan to quit smoking in the near future tend to use smoking to control body weight.(4)

To begin with, let's look at the title of this chapter: "But I Don't Want to Gain Weight!" Who does? Very few people do, except for those who are extremely underweight and report that they can never seem to gain weight. However, don't let this concern with weight gain prevent you from quitting a much worse habit.

Many of the comments about weight gain made by women who smoke are subtle . . . others are not. Have you heard any of the following from some of your smoking friends? Have you ever said any of the following?

"I want to quit smoking, but I don't want to blow up like a balloon."

"A friend of mine recently quit smoking and she gained 30 pounds. Isn't that just as dangerous as smoking?"

"I can't *afford* to stop smoking. I'll have to buy a whole new wardrobe!"

"An eight- to ten-pound weight gain is a dress size!"

Sometimes the comments are even stronger. When we pointed out to one smoker that it would be preferable to gain 5–10 pounds rather than risk dying of cancer or heart disease, her response was: "Yeah. But I'll look *great* in my coffin."

Another told us, in a very take-charge manner: "I would like to stop smoking. But I want to let you know right now that I will stay in the program until I gain three pounds. Then I'm gone."

The first four comments are *very* common. If you are like most women smokers, you have either thought or said something like this. The latter two comments are uncommon, but underscore how important post-cessation weight gain is to many women.

Given these concerns, we provide detailed information here about smoking and body weight. This chapter includes up-to-date and reliable information about whether or not ex-smokers gain weight and, if so, how much? We then discuss which women are particularly at risk for large amounts of post-cessation weight gain. Next, we disclose the latest research on what causes weight gain following cessation and answer a *very* common question women smokers ask: "Shouldn't I smoke instead of gaining a lot of weight? Isn't a lot of weight gain just as dangerous?"

Finally, the last two sections provide important information that will help you evaluate whether or not you should try to prevent the weight gain following smoking cessation. If you don't want to gain weight, we give you some simple strategies for avoiding post-cessation weight gain.

DO WOMEN GAIN WEIGHT FOLLOWING SMOKING CESSATION?

The short answer is "probably." However, when you separate the facts about post-cessation weight gain from the myths, you will be better able to keep that weight gain to a minimum.

The myth of the "one-third statistic"

Perhaps you have heard what we call the "one-third statistic." Many programs and materials actually downplay the significance and amount of weight gain following smoking cessation. These programs and materials tell you that about one-third of people gain weight following smoking cessation, about one-third stay the same, and about one-third actually lose weight. This means, in essence, that two-thirds of all women need not worry about post-cessation weight gain—your weight will either stay the same or you will lose weight!

Given your own personal experience with smoking and body weight, our guess is that you probably know that this statistic can't be correct. Indeed, it is not. When we were summarizing the literature in the late 1980s we found almost a hundred articles on the relationship between smoking and body weight. Of all these, not a single article reported results that were even remotely close to supporting this one-third statistic. A colleague of ours thinks she remembers the origin of this statistic. In a room full of eminent smoking researchers several years ago, the topic of who gains weight following cessation came up. Somebody apparently said, "It has been my experience that about one-third gain weight, one-third stay the same . . . . " Somehow, the statistic caught on (partly, perhaps, because it is so reassuring), even though there were no published data to suggest it was true.

As we have mentioned before, it is our policy to give you all the facts, even if the news isn't particularly good. What we are about to tell you is something you probably already suspected:

most people gain weight when they quit smoking. Somewhere between 70 and 80 percent of smokers gain weight when they quit smoking; the rest stay the same. So weight gain following smoking cessation is quite common, but not inevitable.

How much weight, on average, does a woman gain? While there are many studies in this area, probably the best one was reported by Dr. David Williamson and his colleagues from the Centers for Disease Control. These investigators analyzed data from an initial sample of 14,407 adult men and women. The subjects were followed for ten years. During that time, 959 people quit smoking.

Overall, the results were "good news, bad news." The good news was that average weight gain in those who quit smoking was only about seven pounds or less overall, compared to a 4.1 pound gain for nonsmokers. (It is normal to gain a little weight as we age.) However, the bad news was that women gained more weight than men. Women do have reason to be concerned here. On average, men gained 6.2 pounds while women gained 8.3 pounds.

While women (and men) are concerned with any weight gain, their biggest fear is that they will put on 25 pounds or more, which was expressed by the woman who said she didn't want to "blow up like a balloon". Williamson and his colleagues defined a "major weight gain" as one greater than 28 pounds. The good news is that only 13 percent of women gained more than 28 pounds. Thus, while there *is* a risk for large weight gains, it is relatively rare.

As you would expect, many but not all women gain some weight when they quit smoking. Although the average weight gain is not large, it is still considered troublesome for many women. A small percentage of women are at risk for large amounts of weight.

However, there is another way to look at these statistics. If you look carefully at what smoking is doing to your weight, you don't lose weight when you smoke. In fact, your weight will just stay the same over time. As we mentioned above, it is common for nonsmokers to inch up in their weight over time. We tend to gain a pound or so every three to four years, as we get older. Smoking tends to eliminate this creeping weight. You don't have much, if any, weight gain when you smoke over time; you tend not to gain the normal weight you would have gained.(4) We now know that when you quit smoking, *you merely return to the weight you would have been if you never had smoked!*(5)

The average weight gain for women following smoking cessation is about eight pounds. If you had gained about three to four pounds every 10 years as a nonsmoker, at the end of 20 years you would be six to eight pounds heavier. So, if you stop smoking after 20 years and gain eight pounds, your weight will be where it would have been if you had never smoked. A simple way of looking at this is that smoking keeps your body weight artificially low and this weight gain is your body's way of catching up to where it ought to be.

While all of this makes sense in the abstract, few women think of this as the body catching up when we quit smoking. The weight gain tends to come suddenly and we view it as unnatural because we have never had this weight before. Also, gaining a pound every couple of years seems to be a whole lot easier to take than a rapid eight-pound weight gain. If you are like most women who are quitting smoking, you are still thinking about that 13 percent of women who gain more than 28 pounds and saying to yourself:

"Eight pounds I can take off. I've lost that much before. But 28 pounds . . . that's serious. How do I know if I'm one of the 13 percent that 'blimp out?'"

WHO IS AT RISK FOR EXCESSIVE POST-CESSATION WEIGHT GAIN?

There are some factors that are known to relate to excessive weight gain following smoking cessation. You can evaluate whether your risk for excessive post-cessation weight gain is low or high. This will help you determine what steps, if any, you will take to reduce weight gain.

First, it appears that minorities in general, and African-Americans in particular, are at high risk for post-cessation weight gain. Our research indicates that African-American women gain nearly twice as much weight following smoking cessation as Euroamerican women. Because African-American women are already at high risk for obesity, hypertension, and diabetes, this weight gain is harmful for health. Why it occurs is not known, but it could result from the fact that many African-American women have lower incomes and, consequently, less knowledge of dieting strategies, less access to exercise facilities, and poorer nutrition.

Another factor related to excessive weight gain is how long you have smoked. The longer you have smoked, the more likely it is that you will experience weight gain. By long we mean those who have smoked for over 20 or 30 years. This makes sense if you realize that smoking prevents the normal weight gain associated with growing older (and does not help you lose weight). The longer you smoke, the longer smoking has repressed this weight gain.

Those who smoke heavily (one or more packs a day) are also at higher risk for post-cessation weight gain. This also makes sense. Because nicotine is probably the primary drug responsible for the lowered body weight, the more you smoke, the more nicotine you get. Also, our research found that the metabolic rate—the number of calories you burn at rest—of moderate smokers did not increase following smoking. Only those who smoked heavily had an increase in metabolic rate. This may be why those who smoke heavily gain more weight after stopping.

Interestingly, smokers who are slender or of normal weight are at higher risk for weight gain after quitting than overweight smokers. If you are a bit overweight and are smoking to control your body weight, smoking probably isn't doing you any good!

Our research also confirmed other studies which show that overweight smokers' metabolic rates did not increase when they smoked. Yet there was an increase in the metabolic rate for smokers whose weight was normal. Again, this may explain why normal weight, and not overweight, smokers are at risk for weight gain.

The person who is at particular risk for post-cessation weight gain is an African-American normal-weight smoker who smokes over a pack a day and has smoked for many, many years. Being in a high-risk group does not mean that weight gain is inevitable, it just means that you need to be a bit more vigilant if you want to avoid it. Similarly, we need to be honest and tell you that being in a low-risk group does not mean that you won't necessarily gain any weight—it just means that weight gain is less likely. It may also mean that you will not need to change your lifestyle quite as much if you want to avoid post-cessation weight gain.

WHY DO WOMEN GAIN WEIGHT FOLLOWING SMOKING CESSATION?

Many people assume that all weight gain is related to eating too much. In truth, body weight is determined largely by biochemical, physiological, and genetic processes. Weight gain doesn't necessarily meant that a person is eating more.

There are basically three reasons why people gain weight: they decrease their physical activity, increase their intake of dietary fat, or lower their metabolic rate.

It does not appear that physical activity decreases following smoking cessation. If anything, physical activity may actually increase. Since people often feel better after they quit smoking they may get out more and become more active.

It is also important to note that women (and men) generally do not gain weight by increasing their total caloric intake.(6) They gain weight due to changes in how much fat they eat in their diet. If they increase their fat intake, their weight increases. The implication is that if you just ate less fat you would lose weight! We will discuss this in more detail.

When women quit smoking, it appears that they increase their fat and sugar consumption, at least for a while.(7) When these women return to the eating habits they had when they were smoking, they continue to gain some weight. So increased fat intake appears to explain part, but not all, of the weight gain women experience when they quit smoking.

This leaves metabolic rate. Resting metabolic rate accounts for most of the calories you burn in a day. This is the energy that keeps your body going by maintaining a temperature of 98.6 degrees, taking in oxygen, and pumping your blood. Even a one or two percent shift in resting metabolic rate can put you at risk for a weight gain in a short period of time.

Smoking *does* appear to increase metabolic rate, at least for a short while after smoking. While the increase in metabolic rate doesn't last very long, the number of cigarettes smoked in a day will cause the body to go on a metabolic roller coaster throughout the day. While this in itself may be quite dangerous, it does have the effect of burning calories. However, not all studies find an increase in metabolic rate.(8) We think this is due to the fact that some people experience an increase in metabolic rate when they smoke; others don't. As we mentioned above, we have found that normal-weight smokers and those who smoke heavily generally have an increase in metabolic rate; overweight smokers and those who smoke moderately or lightly do not. We are confident that more studies in this area will help us identify other factors related to metabolic rate as well.

So it appears that metabolic rate can play a significant role in post-cessation weight gain. However, it is important to point out that you will notice an increase of a couple of pounds right away. Many women, especially those who quit during the latter part of their cycle (or during their period), will report a one- to two-pound weight gain in one week. What they do, simply stated, is freak out. They imagine themselves weighing 26–52 pounds more in a year! This early weight gain is probably due to changes in body water. Nicotine is a diuretic, meaning that it tends to clear water out of your system. This apparent rapid weight gain can occur quickly when you quit smoking.

While more studies need to be conducted in this area, be reassured that this rapid weight gain in the first week won't continue. Don't be fooled if you experience an apparent jump in your weight in the first week or so.

"Shouldn't I smoke instead of gaining a lot of weight—isn't a lot of weight gain just as dangerous?"

We hear this excuse (as you will see, it is really a mental gremlin) from many women. If you are truly worried that gaining so much weight will be as unhealthy as smoking, you need not be concerned. The average weight gained by most women does not pose a health risk. Even if someone gained a large amount of weight, as much as 30 pounds, it would not begin to equal the health consequences of smoking.

Many people ask us how much weight gain would be as unhealthy as smoking. This is difficult to say, since everyone is different and it would depend on a number of factors such as your current weight and whether or not you are prone to such diseases as diabetes and high blood pressure. However, many of us in the field estimate that you would have to gain at least 100–150 pounds to equal the health consequences of smoking. If you are concerned about the health risk of gaining weight because of smoking cessation, forget it.

If you are absolutely certain that you do not want to gain weight, use some of our recommended strategies instead of continuing to smoke. Realize that smoking doesn't help you lose weight. While it may help you to maintain your weight, it does so in a detrimental way. Smoking, which is a poison, raises your metabolic rate because your body is trying to get rid of low doses of toxic, potentially lethal agents. Similarly, your metabolism rises—and creates a fever—when you are trying to ward off a viral or bacterial infection. There are many things that raise your metabolic rate that you would find unacceptable: ingesting low doses of rat poison, contracting a virus such as AIDS, or breathing the exhaust from a bus every hour or so. These examples sound extreme and they are . . . but don't fool yourself that you are doing anything different when you smoke. There are *healthy* ways to increase your metabolic rate—exercise, for example.

In Chapter 3 we speculated what an instruction label would look like if the FDA regulated smoking. It is clear that the tobacco companies market cigarettes as a way to control your weight. We imagine that if cigarettes were ever given a truth-in-advertising label, it would look something like this:

"This product has been heavily advertised as a successful weight-loss product. However, regular use of this product will not reduce your weight. Consistent use of this product will prevent the normal one-pound weight gain every three years or so. When use is discontinued, all prevented weight is regained. Warning: This product is highly addictive. If this product were regulated by the Food and Drug Administration, it couldn't even be sold as a prescription medicine. Regular use will shorten your life through a number of diseases that produce slow, painful death."

SHOULD I EVEN BOTHER DOING ANYTHING ABOUT THIS WEIGHT GAIN?

If you are like most women, you are sensitive about your weight. Probably the two most awkward questions people ask us are our age and our weight! So it is not too surprising when we become sensitive regarding post-cessation weight gain. This is illustrated in Garrison Keillor's short story, "The End of the Trail." We used part of this story to illustrate the fact that most people feel that they are among the last few smokers in America. The story has an interesting ending:

> [One reconditioned smoker] was soon reunited with her family, and one night, while crossing a busy intersection near their home in Chicago, she saved them from sure death by pulling them back from the path of a speeding car. Her husband, who had just been telling her she could stand to lose some weight, was killed instantly, however.

Hopefully, most women are not quite *this* sensitive about their weight!

If you are like most women, then you are concerned about weight gain. You may not quit (or you may relapse) if you gain much weight. Again, we can understand this concern, which is why the last section of this chapter provides simple strategies for avoiding the weight gain. Before you take the time and effort to do this, however, ask yourself, "How important is it to me to avoid this weight gain?"

There are four reasons for not worrying about the weight gain and accepting it, particularly if you are currently underweight or normal weight or if you are at a low risk for gaining excessive amounts of weight. First, as we have mentioned above, weight gain is not excessive and almost never poses a health risk for the vast majority of women.

Second, the national obsession with weight control is doing more harm than good. More than twice as many women report they are trying to lose weight than men; two-thirds of women aged 19–39 believe they are overweight.(9) Over the past thirty years, society's concept of what constitutes an ideal body frame has gone from slightly overweight (plump) to near anorexic. Take a look at the ideal body frame thirty years ago. Most people would agree that one of the most attractive women of that time was Marilyn Monroe. Monroe had a full body and, if anything, tended to be just a bit overweight or voluptuous. This body frame was considered highly desirable.

Now look at the ideal bodies of today. While athletic bodies are popular, models today are typically underweight. It has become worse in the last couple of years; it is not uncommon to see "ideal frames" that border on anorexic, with ribs showing.

This zeal for not just normal-weight status but for being thin is an obsession that makes no sense. It is just as unhealthy to be underweight as it is to be overweight. Because weight is carefully regulated by the body, most people's weight loss efforts fail. People go on one diet after another, losing weight, regaining it, going on another diet, regaining it, etc. At a consensus conference on obesity at the National Institutes of Health there was considerable discussion whether this weight cycling, the "yo-yo syndrome" as it is called, may be as physically unhealthy as just being overweight. Typical dieting, which is characterized by losing then regaining weight, may be more physically dangerous than if the person did nothing at all. Unless you are convinced that you really need to avoid this weight gain, you may decide not to buy into this national obsession.

A third reason for accepting this weight gain is that you may be more successful at quitting if you don't also try to maintain or lose weight. People who struggle to gain very little or no weight when they quit smoking may be more likely to relapse than those who accept the weight gain. If you are trying to do two things simultaneously—quit smoking and control your weight—you may become overwhelmed and give up. Also, as we mentioned earlier, smoking is highly reinforcing. So is eating. If you entirely remove one reinforcer *and* greatly curtail another, you may fail at both.(10) It may be easier if you focus on one thing at a time, something we discuss at more length below.

A final reason to consider accepting a few pounds is that you are greatly increasing your physical attractiveness to other people by quitting smoking. As we mentioned in Chapter 3, one study compared interviews with actresses who smoked in one tape but didn't in another. When the actresses smoked, the viewers rated them as less friendly and less moral (more promiscuous). These views were held by males, females, smokers, and nonsmokers alike. A couple of pounds aren't going to stack up to the positive physical image you are going to enjoy by quitting smoking.

For these reasons, we hope you will at least consider focusing your energy on quitting smoking and not concern yourself with the weight gain—at least for a while. On the other hand, if concern about weight gain is very high for you (or you are at high risk for excessive weight gain), we now discuss simple strategies for avoiding post-cessation weight gain. These are also good strategies for weight loss in general.

You now have two options: either quit smoking and don't worry about the weight gain, or quit smoking and decide to make the extra effort to avoid the weight gain. You no longer need to worry about the option you are now using—not quitting for fear of weight gain.

I DON'T WANT TO GAIN WEIGHT— WHAT SHOULD I DO?

There are two reasons why people don't want to gain weight when they quit smoking. The first is that a major weight gain is unhealthy. The second, which we think is much more common, is that they don't want the weight gain for cosmetic reasons—they feel they won't look as physically attractive, won't like themselves as much, or will have to go out and buy new clothes. While many people say they are worried about the health consequences of a large weight gain, we suspect that if they were really honest with themselves, they would acknowledge that they are more concerned about their appearance.

It's okay to feel this way. We can certainly understand that this concern may be preventing you from quitting. But don't let it. If you don't want to gain the weight, you can do something about it. Not quitting should not be an option.

One of the things you can do about it is watch your fat intake. Remember that it is typical for women who quit smoking to begin eating more fat and sugar. You can exert control here. What you won't be able to control is the change in metabolic rate that is likely to occur when you quit smoking. You have gotten used to this abnormally elevated metabolic rate, and may eat a bit more, perhaps, or exercise a bit less than is good for you. A change in metabolic rate does not mean that weight gain is inevitable, however, and we have taken the change in metabolic rate into account in our recommendations below.

What we recommend are changes in lifestyle. Dieting, as we discuss below, won't work. The good news is you do not even have to cut back much on what you eat or do much more exercise to avoid the weight gain. By changing *what* you eat (not how much) and making a few simple changes in your activity patterns, you should be able to reduce or eliminate the unwanted weight gain. We base the following seven simple rules on the latest work at our Prevention Center to help women (smokers and nonsmokers) lose or maintain their weight. These successful strategies are based on our research and the work of eminent scholars across the country.

Wait until you get over the hump of quitting smoking before you make lifestyle changes

As we said before, there is some evidence to suggest that people who gain some weight after they quit smoking are more likely to stay off cigarettes than those who don't gain weight. Perhaps when people try to exercise, change their diet, and quit smoking all at the same time, they are less likely to quit smoking. We recommend that you quit smoking first and feel comfortable with quitting smoking. Wait at least two weeks (preferably a month or more) until the worst of the withdrawal symptoms subside. Then you can channel some of your efforts toward avoiding the weight gain.

Also, recall that nicotine gum and the over-the-counter product phenylpropanolamine (PPA) reduce post-cessation weight gain at least while people are taking these products. If you need longer to get over the effects of quitting smoking, consider the short-term use of these products. If you decide to use nicotine replacement therapy and are concerned about weight gain, you may want to opt for nicotine gum instead of the patch. Regular use of nicotine gum reduces post-cessation weight gain; regular use of the patch does not.

Don't do nothing

Is this your plan for reducing post-cessation weight gain: "Well, you know, I'll watch what I eat—make sure I don't eat any more. And I'll make sure I continue to go three times a week to the health club . . . "?

Many women think that as long as they don't increase their food intake or decrease their activity, they will avoid the post-cessation weight gain. In other words, if they make no changes, they won't gain weight. Since we now know that a large percentage of post-cessation weight gain is caused by your metabolic rate returning to normal, you *will* gain weight if you simply maintain the status quo. Many women who don't understand this get frustrated by their weight gain, because they have watched what they eat and have continued to exercise.

Once your body adjusts to not having poison in it and your metabolic rate normalizes, your body will start needing slightly fewer calories than before, because it will burn less calories. If you want to avoid the weight gain, you need to make a few, simple, permanent changes in your lifestyle.

Don't go on a diet

Perhaps you have seen the woman on television trying to sell her weight loss program by telling you "diets don't work." She is right about that, you know. People think diets are temporary;

something that you go "on" to lose weight and go "off" once the weight is off. The problem is that what people eat when they go off their diet is the very thing that got them over-weight in the first place.

The weight loss industry is clearly in the middle of a crisis. Weight loss programs generally don't work. We feel that one major reason for this (beyond the notion that people use these programs to go "on" and "off" diets) is that these pro-grams have become too complex. We are required to monitor our intake, weigh foods, come to class every week, weigh our-selves a couple of times a week, count calories, and eat certain types of foods. We become so overwhelmed with all the things we are supposed to do that we give up.

If you talk to people who have successfully lost weight on their own, you find that the key to their success was the sim-plicity of their program. They adopted very simple rules, con-sistently adhered to these rules, and continued to use the rules even after they lost the weight. Talk to someone who has lost weight and kept it off and you *won't* hear something like this:

> "Well, I bought four exercise tapes, joined six weight-loss programs, and bought every diet advertised on TV. I weigh and measure all my foods. I only buy foods from one of the diet companies and don't ever eat in restau-rants. I exercise every day and have buns of bronze, tight thighs, and do stomach workouts every day."

Instead, you are likely to hear something like: "I'll tell you what did it for me . . . . " followed by one or at most two short sentences. They tend to be simple things: things that are easy to follow, don't take hours per day, and don't radically alter your daily life. They have done something that is so simple that it is easy to consistently do it for the rest of your life.

Not gaining weight following smoking cessation (or get-ting rid of it) should be approached the same way . . . using simple rules. You don't want to rely on a diet to lose those pounds. You need to make simple, subtle, permanent changes in your lifestyle. Change what you eat, how you eat, and increase your daily activities a bit—in other words, change your lifestyle. Our next three recommendations explain the simple rules you should be following:

Stop counting calories; watch your fat intake

The more we learn about fat, the more we learn that it is bad for us—particularly saturated fat (or fats that are labeled "hydrogenated"). If you can reduce fat to 20–25 percent of your total calorie intake, you will lose weight. You probably won't be able to eat enough of other foods to gain weight if you cut out the fat! Stop counting calories, stop recording what you eat and weighing it. Just cut your fat intake to 20–25 percent of your total intake. A study that looked at weight changes in women smokers and nonsmokers over a two-year period found that the two biggest predictors of change in body weight were the woman's fat intake at the beginning of the study and the amount her fat intake increased over the course of the study. Changes in certain types of activity were also found to be important. However, fat intake was most predictive of weight gain.

Reducing your fat intake helps in other ways as well. Low fat intake is associated with lowered risk of colon and rectal cancer and perhaps breast cancer.(11) Low fat intake reduces cholesterol and is associated with lower risk of heart disease. The American Heart Association, American Dietetics Association, and American Diabetes Association (to name a few) have actively endorsed low-fat diets.

Just stay away from fat. There are a number of books that tell you where the fat is in foods; become a fat detective when you shop. "Low cholesterol" doesn't help in controlling your weight; "no fat" does. Dairy products, such as cheeses and milk (opt for nonfat milk), are full of fat. Many cuts of meat have fat in them, as do most nuts, potato chips, and snacks that tend to be salty. Rich sauces, mayonnaise, and salad dressing are full of fat. If you use a lot of salad dressing you are probably getting more calories from that than from the entire salad. In general, if a food makes your fingers greasy or tends to melt at room temperature, it is probably high in fat. Many things that we think are high in sugar are, in fact, high in fat—including cookies, cakes, pies, ice cream, and candy bars. It's the fat that makes these things taste good, more than the sugar. If you want to taste a snack that is made from all sugar but no fat, try some Gummi Bears. You are much better off eating something with sugar and no fat than something with fat and no sugar. There are good fat substitutes on the market right now and many of these products are excellent. Again, worry only about fat. Remember, use everything in moderation. If you eat enough of anything with calories, it is still theoretically possible to gain weight. However, we think you will be amazed at how easy it is to lose weigh if you just limit your fat intake.

Be sure to read food labels and look for the number of fat grams. Don't buy any food at the supermarket without checking the fat grams. Multiply the grams by nine to find out how many calories from fat are in a single serving. Divide that number by the total calories in a serving and you will know the percentage of fat in the product. Be careful about the calories in a serving. Many food companies, in an attempt to make their product appear less fattening, list serving sizes that barely satisfy the average gerbil. For example, we read a potato chip label that listed a serving size as "three chips." When was the last time any of us ate just three chips?

Change your eating patterns—when you eat and how often

We recommend that people always eat within an hour of rising in the morning and never eat within an hour of going to bed at night. It is common for people who have weight problems to skip breakfast and sometimes lunch. They become so hungry that they wind up eating more when they do eat. The key is to eat a number of small meals and some low-fat snacks. Not only does this keep you from overeating, it keeps your metabolic rate much higher than if you eat less frequently. A higher metabolism means you are burning more calories.

Also, don't eat within an hour of going to bed. Your metabolism normally increases after you have eaten. However, if you go to bed within an hour of eating, your metabolic rate may slow. Remember that you are at high risk for smoking relapse when you are tired. The same thing applies to overeating; your control over eating is less when you are tired. And you are typically the most tired right before you go to bed. So adopt this rule to reduce the probability of late-night binge eating.

Start moving

One thing about people who lose weight and keep it off is clear—virtually all of them increase their physical activity. Contrary to what you may have heard, the best way for people to lose weight may not be to join a health club, go to aerobics every day, or buy and use an exercise bike. If you do these things, or want to do these things, wonderful. However, the best way to lose weight is not to focus on increasing the time spent in aerobic activity but to focus on decreasing the time spent in sedentary (motionless or "couch potato") activities. A study found much higher, long-term weight loss when the exercise program focused on decreasing these sedentary activities. So, stop being a couch potato. Decrease being motionless. Turn off the television. Stand and walk around when you talk on the phone. If you have access to a stationary bike, read while pedaling slowly. Or just change chairs every 15 minutes while reading. We don't care what other types of activities you do—gardening, puttering around the house, jogging, walking, yoga, you name it. In terms of activity, just do less of nothing.

Go out of your way to burn a couple of calories. Walk up one flight of stairs instead of taking the elevator. Park farther away from the shopping mall. Walk from one bus stop to another. It has never ceased to amaze us how people will wait in their cars for a better parking spot for 15 minutes—so they can park closer to their aerobics class!

The key is increasing your activity, just a little bit, many times a day. If you want to start a formal exercise program, all the better. But simply decreasing sedentary activity consistently, and sticking with it, should be enough.

Watch out for one thing. Never use this activity as an excuse for overeating. We have lost count of the number of times people have told us: "I went to aerobics, so I treated myself to a hot fudge sundae." You shouldn't replace the calories you burn by overeating. These simple activities should not become an excuse, or mental gremlin, for eating too much.

If you have already gained weight after you have quit, your weight will start coming off a bit more slowly than if you were on a "crash" diet? But this is the way your body is supposed to lose weight. It is also the way to keep it off.

The poison is in the dose

This means that it isn't bad if you have a high-fat treat every now and then. It is how much and how often that is important. For example, small amounts of alcohol may aid digestion and lower cholesterol. However, large amounts of alcohol can be deadly. Many people think, when they alter their lifestyle, that they should never eat high-fat food again. If this sounds like a mental gremlin, it is. Mental gremlins are as common when trying to lose weight as they are in smoking cessation programs. If you believe that you can never have high-fat food again, never splurge, or never overeat a little again, then this belief may set you up for failure. Unless people have unbelievable amounts of willpower, they will eventually slip and eat a high-fat meal. It is common for people to feel guilty after eating these foods and say to themselves "What's the use?" Then they go back to their old eating habits.

However, if you give yourself permission, every now and then, to have a treat, it makes the treat special. You can save up for this high-fat meal by eating extra carefully the day before or after. You are more likely to continue to eat right if you give yourself permission, every now and then, to have a treat. The key is to have your *average* daily intake from calories be 20–25 percent from fat. If on two days you average 15 percent and on your "treat" day you average 30 percent, this is fine.

Just like the simple rules for relapse, carefully follow these simple rules for avoiding weight gain. You will find that avoiding weight gain is easier than you thought.

THE FINAL STEP

We now come to the end of this book. But for you, it is just a beginning . . . the beginning of a life free from smoking. In this book you have learned many things about what smoking does to you as a woman and how tobacco companies manipulate you for the sole purpose of perpetuating their enormous profits. You know about nicotine replacement options, and when and if to use them. You have learned simple strategies for quitting smoking and avoiding relapse. You know about mental gremlins and how to counteract them. You also know how to deal with the unwanted weight gain when you quit.

The final step is up to you. Only you can decide to quit smoking . . . we have just tried to make it a little easier. You *have* the self-control and willpower to get rid of a habit that you know is killing you. Follow through and keep trying until you succeed. Work at it like you have never worked before, because your life likely depends on it. We know you will enjoy your life without cigarettes. And we wish you the best of luck in the future . . . may it be a long one!

NOTES

U.S. Department of Health and Human Services has been abbreviated to USDHHS, and U.S. Government Printing Office to USGPO, throughout.

Chapter 1

1. American Cancer Society (1986). Women and Smoking. *Healthline* 5, 12–13.

2. USDHHS (1990). *The Health Benefits of Smoking Cessation: Report of the Surgeon General* (DHHS No. CDC 90–8416). Washington DC: USGPO.

3. Ibid.

4. Ibid.

5. Benowitz, N.L. (1990). Clinical Pharmacology of Inhaled Drugs of Abuse: Implications in Understanding Nicotine Dependence. *NIDA Research Monograph* 99, 12–29.

6. Pickworth, W.B., Herning, R.I., and Henningfield, J.E. (1986). Electroencephalographic Effects of Nicotine Chewing Gum in Humans. *Pharmacology, Biochemistry, and Behavior* 25, 879–882.

7. Mishkin, M. and Appenzeller, T. (1987). The Anatomy of Memory. *Scientific American* 256, 80–89.

8. USDHHS (1988). *The Health Consequences of Smoking: Report of the Surgeon General* (DHHS No. 88–8406). Washington DC: USGPO.

9. Hughes, J.R., Gust, S.W., Keenan, R., Fenwick, J.W., Skoo, K., and Higgins, S.T. (1991). Long-term Use of Nicotine vs Placebo Gum. *Archive of Internal Medicine* 151, 1993–1998.

10. USDHHS (1990), Op. cit.

11. Davis, R.M. (1987). Current Trends in Cigarette Advertising and Marketing. *New England Journal of Medicine* 316, 725–732; Flay, B.R. (1987). Mass Media and Smoking Cessation: A Critical Review. *American Journal of Public Health* 77, 153–158; Tye, J.B., Warner, K.E., and Glantz, S.A. (1987). Tobacco Advertising and Consumption: Evidence of a Causal Relationship. *Journal of Public Health Policy* Winter, 492–508.

12. Frazee, L. (1989). *Power Stop*. Fort Collins CO: J.S. Consumer Products.

13. Hughes, J.R. (1992). Smoking: New Direction in Clinical Research. *The Society of Behavioral Medicine Thirteenth Annual Scientific Sessions* 29. [Abstract]

14. Horowitz, M.B., Hindi-Alexander, M., Wagner, T.J. (1985). Psychosocial Mediators of Abstinence, Relapse, and Continued Smoking: A One-Year Follow-up of a Minimal Intervention. *Addictive Behaviors* 10, 29–39.

15. USHDDS (1988), Op. cit.

16. Benowitz, N.L., Hall, S.M., and Modin, G. (1989). Persistent Increase in Caffeine Concentrations in People Who Stop Smoking. *British Medical Journal* 298, 1075–1076.

17. Fisher, E.B., Rehberg, H.R., Beaupre, P.M., Hughes, C.R., Levitt-Gilmore, T., Davis, J.R., and DiLorenzo, T.M. (1991). Gender Differences in Response to Social Support in Smoking Cessation. *Association for Advancement of Behavior Therapy*, November.

18. Benowitz, N.L. and Jacob, P. III. (1984). Daily Intake of Nicotine During Cigarette Smoking. *Clinical Pharmacology and Therapeutics* 35, 499–504.

19. Pirie, P.L., et al. (1991). Gender Differences in Cigarette Smoking and Quitting in a Cohort of Young Adults. *American Journal of Public Health* 81, 324–327.

20. Williamson, D.F., Madans, J., Anda, R.F., Kleinman, J.C., Giovino, G.A., and Byers, T. (1991). Smoking Cessation and Severity of Weight Gain in a National Cohort. *New England Journal of Medicine* 324 (11), 739–745.

21. Curry, S.J., Marlatt, G.A., Gordon, J.R., and Baer, J.S. (1988). A Comparison of Alternative Theoretical Approaches to Smoking Cessation and Relapse. *Health Psychology* 7, 545–556.

Chapter 2

1. Mattson, M.E., et al. (1987). What Are the Odds That Smoking Will Kill You? *American Journal of Public Health* 77, 425–431.

2. U.S. Environmental Protection Agency (1992). *Respiratory Health Effects of Passive Smoking: Lung Cancer and Other Disorders*. Washington DC: U.S. EPA.

3. Burchfiel, C.M., et al. (1986). Passive Smoking in Children: Respiratory Conditions and Pulmonary Function in Tecumseh, Michigan. *American Review of Respiratory Diseases* 133, 966–973.

4. Reed, B.D., and Lutz, L.J. (1988). Household Smoking Exposure: Association with Middle Ear Effusions. *Family Medicine* 20, 426–430.

5. Hoffman, H.J., et al. (1988). Risk Factors for SIDS: Results of the National Institute of Child Health and Human Development SIDS Cooperative Epidemiological Study. *Annals of the New York Academy of Sciences* 533, 13–29.

6. Moss, A.J., Allen, K.F., Giovino, G.A., Mills, S.L. (1992). Recent Trends in Adolescent Smoking, Smoking Uptake Correlates, and Expectations About the Future. Advance data from vital and health statistics, No. 221. Hyattsville MD: National Center for Health Statistics.

7. Hankinson, S.E., et al. (1992). A Prospective Study of Cigarette Smoking and Risk of Cataract Surgery in Women. *Journal of the American Medical Association* 268, 994–998.

8. Allen, H.B., Johnson, B.L., Diamond, S.M. (1973). Smoker's wrinkles. *Journal of the American Medical Association* 225, 1067–1069.

9. Campbell, O.M. and Gray, R.H. (1987). Smoking and Ectopic Preg-

nancy: A Multinational Case-Control Study. In Rosenberg, M.J. (ed.), *Smoking and Reproductive Health*. Littleton MA: PSG Publishing.

10. USDHHS (1990). *The Health Benefits of Smoking Cessation: Report of the Surgeon General* (DHHS No. CDC 90–8416). Washington DC: USGPO.

11. Schols, D., Daling, J.R., Stergachis, A.S. (1992). Current Cigarette Smoking and Risk of Acute Pelvic Inflammatory Disease. *American Journal of Public Health* 82, 1352–1355.

12. Williams, A.R., Weiss, N.S., Ure, C.L. (1982). Effect of Weight, Smoking, and Estrogen Use on the Risk of Hip and Forearm Fracture in Postmenopausal Women. *Obstetrics and Gynecology* 60, 695–699.

13. Willett, W., et al. (1983). Cigarette Smoking, Relative Weight and Menopause. *American Journal of Epidemiology* 117, 651–658.

14. Kleinman, J.C., et al. (1988). The Effects of Maternal Smoking on Fetal and Infant Mortality. *American Journal of Epidemiology* 126, 274–282.

15. Underwood, P.B., et al. (1967). Parental Smoking Empirically Related to Pregnancy Outcome. *Obstetrics and Gynecology* 29, 1–8.

16. Kleinman, J.C., and Madans, J.H. (1985). The Effects of Maternal Smoking, Physical Stature, and Educational Attainment on the Incidence of Low Birth Weight. *American Journal of Epidemiology* 121, 843–855; Rush, D. and Cassano, P. (1983). Relationship of Cigarette Smoking and Social Class to Birth Weight and Perinatal Mortality Among All Births. *Journal of Epidemiology and Community Health* 37, 249–255; USDHHS, Op. cit.

17. USDHHS, Op. cit.

18. Ibid.

19. Kristein, M. (1982). *The Economics of Health Promotion at a Worksite.* New York: American Health Foundation.

20. Bilheimer, D.W. (1988). Therapeutic Control of Hyperlipidemia in the Prevention of Coronary Atherosclerosis: A Review of Results from Recent Clinical Trials. *American Journal of Cardiology* 62, 1J–9J.

21. USDHHS (1988). *The Health Consequences of Smoking: Report of the Surgeon General* (DHHS No. 88–8406). Washington DC: USGPO.

22. Mattson, et al., Op. cit.

23. Ibid.; USDHHS (1990), Op. cit.

Chapter 3

1. Federal Trade Commission (1985). *Report to Congress Pursuant to the Federal Cigarette Labeling and Advertising Act for the Years 1982–1983.* June 1985. Washington DC: Federal Trade Commission.

2. USDHHS (1989). *Requirements of Laws and Regulations Enforced by the U.S. Food and Drug Administration.* USDHHS, Public Health Service, Food and Drug Administration, Office of Public Affairs. (DHHS No. FDA 89–1115).

3. Davis, R.M. (1987). Current Trends in Cigarette Advertising and Marketing. *New England Journal of Medicine* 316, 725–732.

4. Tye, J.B., Warner, K.E., and Glantz, S.A. (1987). Tobacco Advertising and Consumption: Evidence of a Causal Relationship. *Journal of Public Health Policy* Winter, 492–508.

5. Boddewyn, J.J. (1986). Tobacco Advertising in a Free Society. In R.D. Tollison (ed.), *In Smoking and Society: Toward a More Balanced Assessment.* Lexington MA: D.C. Heath and Co.

6. Tye, et al., Op. cit.

7. USHDDS, Op. cit.

8. Davis, Op. cit.

9. Boddewyn, Op. cit.; R.J. Reynolds Tobacco Co. (1984). We Don't Advertise to Children. *Time Magazine* April 9, p. 91.

10. Hutchings, R. (1981). *A Review of the Nature and the Extent of Cigarette Advertising in the United States.* In proceedings of the National Conference on Smoking and Health. New York: American Cancer Society, 241–262; Gorog, W.F. (1986). *Oversight Hearings on Tobacco Advertising.* Subcommittee on Health and the Environment, Committee on Commerce, U.S. House of Representatives, August 1, 1986.

11. Goldstein, A.O., et al. (1987). Relationship Between High School Student Smoking and Recognition of Cigarette Advertisements. *Journal of Pediatrics*, 110, 488–491.

12. Fischer, P.M. et al. (1991). Brand Logo Recognition by Children Aged 3 to 6 Years: Mickey Mouse and Old Joe the Camel. *Journal of the American Medical Association* 266, 3145–3148.

13. DiFranza, J.R. et al. (1991). RJR Nabisco's Cartoon Camel Promotes Camel Cigarettes to Children. *Journal of the American Medical Association* 266, 3149–3153.

14. DiFranza, J.R., and McAfee, T. (1992). The Tobacco Institute: Helping Youth Say "Yes" to Tobacco. *Journal of Family Practice* 34, 694–696.

15. Warner, K.E., et al. (1992). Cigarette Advertising and Magazine Coverage of the Hazards of Smoking: A Statistical Analysis. *New England Journal of Medicine* 326, 305–309.

16. Benowitz, N.L., Jacob, P. III., Kozlowski, L. and Yu, L. (1986). Influence of Smoking Fewer Cigarettes on Exposure to Tar, Nicotine, and Carbon Monoxide Exposure. *New England Journal of Medicine* 314, 1310–1313.

Chapter 4

1. Hughes, J.R. (1991). Combined Psychological and Nicotine Gum Treatment for Smoking: A Critical Review. *Journal of Substance Abuse* 3, 337–350; Transdermal Nicotine Study Group (1991). Transdermal Nicotine for Smoking Cessation: Six-Month Results from Two Multicenter Controlled Clinical Trials. *Journal of the American Medical Association* 266, 3133–3138.

2. Klesges, R.C., Klesges, L.M., Meyers, A.W., Klem, M., and Isbell, T. (1990). The Effects of Phenylpropanolamine on Dietary Intake, Physical Activity, and Body Weight Following Smoking Cessation. *Clinical Pharmacology and Therapeutics* 47, 747–754; Klesges, R.C., Klesges, L.M., Isbell, T.R.,

Klem, M.L., DeBon, M., and Shuster, M.L., (1992). The Effects of Phenyl-propanolamine on Symptoms Associated with Smoking Withdrawal. *Proceedings of the 13th Annual Convention of the Society of Behavioral Medicine*, 103. [Abstract]

3. Glassman, A.H., et al. (1984). Cigarette Craving, Smoking Withdrawal and Clonidine. *Science* 226, 864–866; Ornish, S.A., Zisook, S., and McAdams, L.A. (1988). Effects of Transdermal Clonidine Treatment on Withdrawal Symptoms Associated with Smoking Cessation. *Archives of Internal Medicine* 320, 898–903.

4. USHDDS (1988). *The Health Consequences of Smoking: Report of the Surgeon General* (DHHS No. 88–8406). Washington DC: USGPO.

5. Hughes (1991), Op. cit.; Kottke, T.E., Battista, R.N., DeFriese, G.H., and Brekke, M.L. (1988). Attributes of Successful Smoking Cessation Interventions in Medical Practice: A Meta-analysis of 39 Controlled Trials. *Journal of the American Medical Association* 259, 2882–2889; Daughton, D.M., et al. (1991). Effect of Transdermal Nicotine Delivery as an Adjunct to Low-intervention Smoking Cessation Therapy. A Randomized, Placebo-controlled, Double-Blind Study. *Archives of Internal Medicine* 151, 749–752; Tonnesen, P., Norregaard, J., Simonsen, K., and Sawe, U. (1991). A Double-Blind Trial of a 16-hour Transdermal Nicotine Patch in Smoking Cessation. *New England Journal of Medicine* 325, 311–315; Transdermal Nicotine Study Group, Op. cit.

6. USDHHS, Op. cit.

7. USDHHS (1979). *Smoking and Health: Report of the Surgeon General.* (DHHS No. 79-50066). Washington DC: USGPO; Burns, D.M. (1991) Cigarettes and Smoking. *Clinical Chest Med* 12, 631–642.

8. USDHHS, Op. cit.

9. Ibid.

10. Ibid.

11. Hughes, J.R., Gust, S.W., Keenan, R., Fenwick, J.W., Skoog, K., and Higgins, S.T. (1991) Long-term Use of Nicotine vs Placebo Gum. *Archive of Internal Medicine* 151, 1993–1998.

12. Ibid.

13. USDHHS (1990). *The Health Benefits of Smoking Cessation: Report of the Surgeon General* (DHHS No. CDC 90–8416). Washington DC: USGPO.

14. Benowitz, N.L. and Jacob, P. III (1984). Daily Intake of Nicotine During Cigarette Smoking. *Clinical Pharmacology and Therapeutics* 35, 499–504; Kozlowski, L.T., Fracher, R.C., and Lei, H. (1982). Nicotine Yields of Cigarettes: Plasma Nicotine Levels in Smokers and Public Health. *Preventive Medicine* 11, 240–244.

15. Daughton, et al., Op. cit.; Hughes, Op. cit.; Tonnesen, et al., Op. cit.

16. Transdermal Nicotine Study Group, Op. cit.

17. Klesges, R.C., and Klesges, L.M. (1988). Cigarette Smoking as a Dietary Strategy in a University Population. *International Journal of Eating Disorders* 7, 413–419.

18. USDHHS (1990), Op. cit.; Henningfield, J.E., et al. (1990). Drinking Coffee and Carbonated Beverages Blocks Absorption of Nicotine from Nicotine Polacrilex Gum. *Journal of the American Medical Association* 264, 1560–1564.

Chapter 5

1. Becker, M.H., and Maiman, L.A. (1975). Sociobehavioral Determinants of Compliance with Health and Medical Care Recommendations. *Medical Care* 13, 10–24.

2. Prochaska, J.O. and DiClemente, C.C. (1983). Stages and Processes of Self-change of Smoking: Toward an Integrative Model of Change. *Journal of Consulting and Clinical Psychology* 51, 390–395.

3. Prochaska, J.O. and DiClemente, C.C. (1986). The Transtheoretical Approach: Towards a Systemic Eclectic Framework. In J.C. Norcross (ed.) *Handbook of Eclectic Psychotherapy*. New York: Brunner/Mazel.

4. Curry, S.J., Marlatt, G.A., Gordon, J.R., and Baer, J.S. (1988). A Comparison of Alternative Theoretical Approaches to Smoking Cessation and Relapse. *Health Psychology* 7, 545–556.

5. Fisher, E.B., Rehberg, H.R., Beaupre, P.M., Hughes, C.R., Levitt-Gilmore, T., Davis, J.R., and DiLorenzo, T.M. (1991). Gender Differences in Response to Social Support in Smoking Cessation. *Association for Advancement of Behavior Therapy*, November.

6. Coppotelli, H.C. and Orleans, C.T. (1985). Partner Support and Other Determinants of Smoking Cessation Maintenance Among Women. *Journal of Consulting and Clinical Psychology* 53, 455–460.

7. Lichtenstein, E., Glasgow, R.E., and Abrams, D.B. (1986). Social Support in Smoking Cessation: In Search of Effective Interventions. *Behavior Therapy* 17, 607–619.

8. Coppotelli, H.C., and Orleans, C.T. (1985).

9. USDHHS (1988). *The Health Consequences of Smoking: Report of the Surgeon General* (DHHS No. 88-8406). Washington DC: USGPO.

Chapter 6

1. USDHHS (1990). *The Health Benefits of Smoking Cessation: Report of the Surgeon General* (DHHS No. CDC 90-8416). Washington DC: USGPO.

2. Hughes, J.R., Gust, S.W., Keenan, R., Fenwick, J.W., Skoog, K., and Higgins, S.T. (1991). Long-term Use of Nicotine vs Placebo Gum. *Archive of Internal Medicine* 151, 1993–1998.

Chapter 7

1. Nolen-Hoeksema, S. (1987). Sex Differences in Unipolar Depression: Evidence and Theory. *Psychological Bulletin* 101, 259–282.

2. Kohlberg, L. (1966). A Cognitive-Developmental Analysis of Children's Sex-Role Concepts and Attitudes. In E.E. Maccoby (ed.), *The Development of Sex Differences*. Stanford CA: Stanford University Press.

3. Meichenbaum, D. (1977). *Cognitive Behavioral Modification*. New York: Plenum Publishing.

4. Klesges, R.C. and Klesges, L.M. (1988). Cigarette Smoking as a Dieting Strategy in a University Population. *International Journal of Eating Disorders* 7, 413–419.

5. USDHHS (1990). The Health Benefits of Smoking Cessation: Report of the Surgeon General (DHHS No. CDC 90–8416). Washington DC: US-GPO.

6. Ibid.

Chapter 8

1. USDHHS (1990). *The Health Benefits of Smoking Cessation: Report of the Surgeon General* (DHHS No. CDC 90–8416). Washington DC: USGPO.

2. Shiffman, S. (1982). Relapse Following Smoking Cessation: A Situational Analysis. *Journal of Consulting and Clinical Psychology* 50, 71–86.

3. Marlatt, G.A., and Gordon, J.R. (1985). *Relapse Prevention: Maintenance Strategies in the Treatment of Addictive Behaviors*. New York: Guilford.

4. Carmody, T.P. (1990). Preventing Relapse in the Treatment of Nicotine Addiction: Current Issues and Future Directions. *Journal of Psychoactive Drugs* 22, 211–238.

5. Hymowitz, N. et al. (1991). Baseline Factors Associated with Smoking Cessation and Relapse: MRFIT Group Research. *Preventive Medicine* 20, 590–601.

6. USDHHS (1988). *The Health Consequences of Smoking: Report of the Surgeon General*. (DHHS No. 88-8406). Washington DC: USGPO.

7. Abrams, D.B., et al. (1987). Psychosocial Stress and Coping in Smokers Who Relapse or Quit. *Health Psychology* 6, 289–303.

8. Marlatt and Gordon, Op. cit.

9. Boddewyn, J.J. (1986). Tobacco Advertising in a Free Society. In R.D. Tollison (ed.), *In Smoking and Society: Toward a More Balanced Assessment*. Lexington MA: D.C. Heath and Co.

Chapter 9

1. Sorensen, G. and Pechacek, T.F. (1987). Attitudes Toward Smoking Cessation Among Men and Women. *Journal of Behavioral Medicine* 10, 129–137.

2. Camp, D.E., et al. (1993). The Relationship Between Body Weight Concerns and Adolescent Smoking. *Health Psychology* 12, 24–32.

3. Weekley, C.K., Klesges, R.C., and Relyea, G. (1993). Smoking as a Weight Control Strategy and Its Relationship to Smoking Status. *Addictive Behaviors* 17, 259–271.

4. Klesges, R.C., Meyers, A.W., Klesges, L.M., and LaVasque, M.E. (1989). Smoking, Body Weight, and Their Effects on Smoking Behavior: A Comprehensive Review of the Literature. *Psychological Bulletin* 106, 1–27.

5. Klesges, R.C., Klesges, L.M., and Meyers, A.W. (1991). The Relationship of Smoking Status, Energy Balance, and Body Weight: Analysis of NHANES II. *Journal of Consulting and Clinical Psychology* 59, 899–905.

6. Klesges, R.C., Klesges, L.M., Haddock, C.K., and Eck, L.H. (1992). A Longitudinal Analysis of the Impact of Dietary Intake and Physical Activity on Weight Change in Adults. *American Journal of Clinical Nutrition* 54, 818–822.

7. Hall, S.M. et al. (1989). Changes in Food Intake and Activity After Quitting Smoking. *Journal of Consulting and Clinical Psychology* 57, 81–86.

8. USDHHS (1990). *The Health Benefits of Smoking Cessation: Report of the Surgeon General* (DHHS No. CDC 90–8416). Washington DC: USGPO.

9. National Center for Health Statistics (1985). Provisional data from the Health Promotion and Disease Prevention supplement to the National Health Survey advance data, November 2–5.

10. Epstein, L.H., Bulik C.M., Perkins, K.A., Caggiula, A.R., et al. (1991). Behavioral Economic Analysis of Smoking: Money and Food as Alternatives. *Pharmacology, Biochemistry, and Behavior* 38, 715–791.

11. USDHHS (1988). *The Surgeon General Report on Nutrition and Health*. (DHHS No. 88–50210). Washington, DC: USGPO.

GENERAL REFERENCES

Chapter 1

Benowitz, N.L., Hall, S.M., and Modin, G. (1989). Persistent Increase in Caffeine Concentrations in People Who Stop Smoking. *British Medical Journal* 298, 1075–1076.

Conway, T.L., Vickers, R.R., Ward, H.W., and Rahe, R.H. (1981). Occupational Stress and Variation in Cigarette, Coffee, and Alcohol Consumption. *Journal of Health and Social Behavior* 22, 155–165.

Dirth, C.D. (1971). Smoking Behavior and Its Relation to the Smokers' Immediate Experience. *British Journal of Social and Clinical Psychology* 10, 73–78.

Fisher, E.B., Rehberg, H.R., Beaupre, P.M., Hughes, C.R., Levitt-Gilmore, T., Davis, J.R., and DiLorenzo, T.M. (1991). Gender Differences in Response to Social Support in Smoking Cessation. *Association for Advancement of Behavior Therapy*, November.

Ikard, F.F. and Tomkins, S. (1973). The Experience of Affect as a Determinant of Smoking Behavior: A Series of Validity Studies. *Journal of Abnormal Psychology* 81, 172–181.

Keillor, G. (1989). End of the Trail. In *We Are Still Married*. New York: Dutton.

Livson, N. and Leino, E.V. (1988). Cigarette Smoking Motives: Factorial Structure and Gender Differences in a Longitudinal Study. *The International Journal of Addictions* 23, 535–544.

Shiffman, S. (1986). A Cluster-Analytic Classification of Smoking Relapse Episodes. *Addictive Behaviors* 11, 295–307.

Williamson, D.F., Madans, J., Anda, R.F., Kleinman, J.C., Giovino, G.A., and Byers, T. (1991). Smoking Cessation and Severity of Weight Gain in a National Cohort. *New England Journal of Medicine* 324 (11).

Chapter 2

Hebel, J.R., Fox, N.L., and Sexton, M. (1988). Dose-Response of Birth Weight to Various Measures of Maternal Smoking During Pregnancy. *Journal of Clinical Epidemiology* 41, 483–489.

Physicians' Desk Reference, 44th Edition. (1990). Oradell NJ: Medical Economics Co.

USDHHS (1989). *Reducing and Health Consequences of Smoking: 25 Years of Progress: Report of the Surgeon General.* Public Health Service, Office on Smoking and Health, Rockville, MD.

Chapter 3

Elliott, S. (1988). Marketline: Cigarette Stocks Fall on Liability Verdict. *USA Today,* June 15th, 1988, p. 4B.

Federal Trade Commission (1984). *Report to Congress Pursuant to the Federal Cigarette Labeling and Advertising Act 1984.* Washington DC: FTC. July 1986.

Isbell, T.R., and Klesges, R.C. (1992). Advertising and Smoking Rates in Women and Minorities. Proceedings of the Society of Behavioral Medicine 13th Annual Scientific Sessions, pg. 104.

Klesges, R.C., and Klesges, L.M. (1988). Cigarette Smoking as a Dietary Strategy in a University Population. *International Journal of Eating Disorders* 7, 413–419.

Parry, J. (1987). Fashion Smokes Glow in Switzerland. *Advertising Age* October 12, 1987, p. 68.

Tipper, H. (1988). *Advertising, Its Principles and Practice.* New York: Garland Press.

Tobacco Institute (1987). *Tobacco: Helping Youth Say No.* Washington DC: Tobacco Institute.

USDHHS (1989). *Smoking, Tobacco, and Health: A Fact Book.* USDHHS, Public Health Service, Centers for Disease Control, Center for Chronic Disease Prevention and Health Promotion, Office on Smoking and Health. (DHHS No. CDC 87–8397). Washington DC: USGPO.

Chapter 4

Burns, D.M. (1991). Cigarettes and Cigarette Smoking. *Clinical Chest Med* 12, 631–642.

Hughes, J.R., et al. (1986). Prevalence of Smoking Among Psychiatric Outpatients. *American Journal of Psychiatry* 143, 993–997.

Nolen-Hoeksema, S. (1987). Sex Differences in Unipolar Depression: Evidence and Theory. *Psychological Bulletin* 101, 259–282.

Palmer, K.J., et al. (1992). Transdermal Nicotine: A Review of Its Pharmacodynamic and Pharmacokinetic Properties, and Therapeutic Efficacy As an Aid to Smoking Cessation. *Drugs* 44, 498–529.

Physicians' Desk Reference, 44th edition. (1990). Oradell, NJ: Medical Economics Co.

Rosenstock, I.M. (1992). Patients' Compliance with Health Regimens. *Journal of the American Medical Association* 234, 402–403.

Waal-Manning, H.J. and de Hamel, F.A. (1978) Smoking Habit and Psychometric Scores: A Community Study. *New Zealand Medical Journal* 88, 188–191.

Wager-Srdar, S.A., et al. (1990). Effects of Cigarette Smoke and Nicotine on Feeding and Energy. *Physiology and Behavior* 32, 389–95.

Chapter 5

Hughes, J.R., Gust, S.W., Keenan, R., Fenwick, J.W., Skoog, K., and Higgins, S.T. (1991) Long-term Use of Nicotine vs Placebo Gum. *Archive of Internal Medicine* 151, 1993–1998.

Kohlberg, L. (1966). A Cognitive-Developmental Analysis of Children's Sex-Role Concepts and Attitudes. In E.E. Maccoby (ed.), *The Development of Sex Differences*. Stanford CA: Stanford University Press.

Prochaska, J.O. and DiClemente, C.C. (1986). The Transtheoretical Approach: Towards a Systemic Eclectic Framework. In J.C. Norcross (ed.) *Handbook of Eclectic Psychotherapy*. New York: Brunner/Mazel.

USDHHS. (1990). *The Health Benefits of Smoking Cessation: Report of the Surgeon General*. (DHHS No. CDC 90–8416). Washington DC: USGPO.

Chapter 7

Burns, D.D. (1989). *The Feeling Good Handbook*. New York: Penguin Group.

USDHHS (1988). *The Health Consequences of Smoking: Report of the Surgeon General*. (DHHS No. 88–8406). Washington DC: USGPO.

Chapter 9

Brownell, K.D. (1991). Dieting and the Search for the Perfect Body: Where Physiology and Culture Collide. *Behavior Therapy* 22, 1–12.

Brownell, K.D. and Jeffrey, R.W. (1987). Improving Long-term Weight Loss: Pushing the Limits of Treatment. *Behavior Therapy* 18, 353–374.

Clark, E.M., Klesges, R.C., and Neimeyer, R.A. (1992). Attributions About Sexual Behavior, Attractiveness, and Health as a Function of Subjects' and Targets' Sex and Smoking Status. *Basic and Applied Social Psychology* 13, 205–216.

Cornoni-Huntley, et al. (1989). Race and Sex Differentials in the Impact of Hypertension in the United States. *Archives of Internal Medicine* 149, 780–788.

Hall, S.M., Ginsberg, D., and Jones, R.T. (1986). Smoking Cessation and Weight Gain. *Journal of Consulting and Clinical Psychology* 54, 342–346.

Jequier, E. (1987). Energy Utilization in Human Obesity. In R.J. and J.J. Wurtman (eds.), *Human Obesity*, 73–83. New York: New York Academy of Sciences.

Klesges, R.C., Klesges, L.M., Meyers, A.W., Klem, M., and Isbell, T. (1990). The Effects of Phenylpropanolamine on Dietary Intake, Physical Activity, and Body Weight Following Smoking Cessation. *Clinical Pharmacology and Therapeutics* 47, 747–754.

Pi-Sunyer, F.X. (1990). Obesity and Diabetes in Blacks. *Diabetes Care* 13, 1144–1149.

Rodin, J. (1987). Weight Changes Following Smoking Cessation: The Role of Food Intake and Exercise. *Addictive Behaviors* 12, 303–317.

Schacter, S. (1982). Recidivism and Self-cure of Smoking and Obesity. *American Psychologist* 37, 436–444.

USDHHS (1988). *The Health Consequences of Smoking: Report of the Surgeon General* (DHHS No. 88–8406). Washington DC: USGPO.

USDHHS (1990). *The Health Benefits of Smoking Cessation: Report of the Surgeon General* (DHHS No. CDC 90–8416). Washington DC: USGPO.

Williamson, D.F., Madans, J., Anda, R.F., Kleinman, J.C., Giovino, G.A., and Byers, T. (1991). Smoking Cessation and Severity of Weight Gain in a National Cohort. *New England Journal of Medicine* 324, 739–745.

INDEX

Other Health Books for Women

WOMEN'S CANCERS: How to Prevent Them, How to Treat Them, How to Beat Them by Kerry A. McGinn, R.N. and Pamela J. Haylock, R.N.

Women's Cancers is the first book to focus specifically on the cancers that affect exclusively women—breast, cervical, pelvic, ovarian, uterine, and other rare cancers—offering the latest information from the health care community. The book approaches the subject in a clear, information-driven style, and describes successful prevention, detection, and cancer treatment options in detail. It discusses all the issues, from the psychological to the practical, surrounding a cancer diagnosis.

"WOMEN'S CANCERS is fully comprehensive, helpful to patients and healthcare workers alike. Recommended." — **LIBRARY JOURNAL**

448 pages ... 54 illustrations ... Paperback $14.95 ... Hardcover $24.95

MENOPAUSE WITHOUT MEDICINE by Linda Ojeda, Ph.D., Revised Second Edition

This popular book debunks many of the myths of menopause and provides comprehensive guidelines on holistic, natural ways to prepare for menopause and effectively treat common complaints. The author maintains that good lifestyle habits can make the difference for a carefree menopause, and discusses the impact personal appearance, sexuality, and energy level can have on overall physical and emotional well-being. A new chapter on breast cancer describes risk factors, possible environmental causes, and the important role diet plays in beating cancer.

304 pages ... Paperback ... Second Edition ... $12.95

GETTING PREGNANT AND STAYING PREGNANT: Overcoming Infertility and Managing Your High-Risk Pregnancy by Diana Raab, B.S., R.N.

A complete, accessible, and practical guide to the physical and emotional problems encountered during infertility and high-risk pregnancy. Fully updated with the most current medical information, it describes causes, symptoms, and possible treatments. The author discusses her personal experiences and gives information on such topics as: infertility testing, Cesarean birth, miscarriage, premature birth, nutrition, and new technology.

336 pages ... 28 illustrations ... Paperback ... $12.95

To order please see last page

The A-to-Z Women's Health Series

THE NEW A-TO-Z OF WOMEN'S HEALTH
by Christine Ammer

An up-to-date work that covers all aspects of a woman's health with over 1000 expert entries. A cross-reference system and subject guide that make it easy to use for women and professionals. It discusses timely and important women's health topics, including: pregnancy, childbirth, and birth control * drugs, medication, fitness, and vitamins * cholesterol and diet * chronic disease, disabilities, and surgery * sexuality and sexually transmitted diseases.

"The coverage is more extensive than that of *The New Our Bodies, Ourselves* and more current than that of Felicia Stewart's *Understanding Your Body.*" — BOOKLIST

496 pages ... 10 illustrations ... Paperback ... $16.95

THE A-TO-Z OF WOMEN'S SEXUALITY
by Ada P. Kahn and Linda Hughey Holt, M.D.

This sensitively written book sorts out the information on women's sexuality in a clear, jargon-free style. With over 2000 alphabetically arranged entries, this resource has cross-referenced entries on subjects such as: sexual fears and disorders * the symptoms and complications of sexually transmitted diseases, including AIDS, PID, and chlamydia * female and male sexual response cycles * gynecological tests, medications, and contraception methods.

"Easy to use. An ambitious attempt to compile a vocabulary of sexuality for a popular audience. The wide-ranging interdisciplinary coverage make it a good addition for ready reference." — BOOKLIST

368 pages ... 19 illustrations ... Paperback ... $14.95

THE A-TO-Z OF PREGNANCY AND CHILDBIRTH
by Nancy Evans

This book is a valuable aid for women who are—or plan to be—pregnant. It answers the questions of expectant parents and offers insight into the medical issues and language surrounding pregnancy and childbirth. It has more than 850 clear definitions discussing issues such as: infertility treatments and reproductive technology * breastfeeding and its affects on mother and baby * the controversy over home vs. hospital births. *Includes a special pull-out illustrated chart that tracks monthly fetal and maternal development.*

416 pages ... 16 illustrations ... Paperback $16.95 ... Hardcover $29.95

For our FREE catalog of books
please call 510-865-5282

ORDER FORM

10% DISCOUNT on orders of $20 or more —
20% DISCOUNT on orders of $50 or more —
30% DISCOUNT on orders of $250 or more —
On cost of books for fully prepaid orders

NAME

ADDRESS

CITY/STATE   ZIP

COUNTRY [outside USA]   POSTAL CODE

TITLE	QTY	PRICE	TOTAL
A-to-Z of Pregnancy and Childbirth *(pb)*	|	@ $ 16.95	
A-to-Z of Pregnancy and Childbirth *(hc)*	|	@ $ 29.95	
(New) A-to-Z of Women's Health	|	@ $ 16.95	
A-to-Z of Women's Sexuality	|	@ $ 14.95	
Getting Pregnant and Staying Pregnant	|	@ $ 12.95	
How Women Can *Finally* Stop Smoking	|	@ $ 8.95	
Menopause Without Medicine	|	@ $ 12.95	
Women's Cancers *(paperback)*	|	@ $ 14.95	
Women's Cancers *(hardcover)*	|	@ $ 24.95	

Shipping costs:
First book: $2.50
($3.50 for Canada)
Each additional book:
$.75 ($1.00 for
Canada)
For UPS rates and
bulk orders call us at
(510) 865-5282

TOTAL	
Less discount @_____%	(_____)
TOTAL COST OF BOOKS	_____
Calif. residents add sales tax	_____
Shipping & handling	_____
TOTAL ENCLOSED	══════
Please pay in U.S. funds only	

❑ Check   ❑ Money Order   ❑ Visa   ❑ M/C

Card # _____ Exp date _____

Signature _____

Complete and mail to

Hunter House Inc., Publishers
PO Box 2914, Alameda CA 94501-0914
Phone (510) 865-5282 Fax (510) 865-4295
❑ Check here to receive our book catalog

HOW 12/93